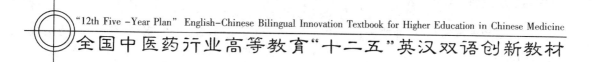
Processing of Chinese Materia Medica

中 药 炮 制 学

（英汉对照）

（English – Chinese）

Editor – in – Chief　Zhong Lingyun，David Karlau，Gong Qianfeng

主　编　钟凌云　戴维·卡劳（美）　龚千锋

China Press of Traditional Chinese Medicine

中国中医药出版社

· Beijing ·

· 北 京 ·

图书在版编目（CIP）数据

中药炮制学：英汉对照/钟凌云，（美）卡劳，龚千锋主编.—北京：中国中医药出版社，2015.3

全国中医药行业高等教育"十二五"英汉双语创新教材

ISBN 978 - 7 - 5132 - 2399 - 7

Ⅰ.①中… Ⅱ.①钟… ②卡… ③龚… Ⅲ.①中药炮制学 - 双语教学 - 中医药院校 - 教材 - 英、汉 Ⅳ.①R283

中国版本图书馆 CIP 数据核字（2015）第 025750 号

中国中医药出版社出版

北京市朝阳区北三环东路 28 号易亨大厦 16 层

邮政编码　100013

传真　010 64405750

北京泰锐印刷有限公司印刷

各地新华书店经销

*

开本 787×1092　1/16　印张 14.5　字数 525 千字

2015 年 3 月第 1 版　2015 年 3 月第 1 次印刷

书　号　ISBN 978 - 7 - 5132 - 2399 - 7

*

定价　30.00 元

网址　www.cptcm.com

全国中医药行业高等教育"十二五"英汉双语创新教材

《中药炮制学》（英汉对照）编委会

"12th Five – Year Plan" English – Chinese Bilingual Innovation
Textbook for Higher Education in Chinese Medicine

Processing of Chinese Materia Medica（English – Chinese）

Editorial Board

编写说明

中药炮制是我国独有的制药技术，通过炮制加工的中药饮片，与中药材、中成药并称为中药产业的三大支柱。围绕中药炮制技术建立的中药炮制学学科是我国中医药学科重要的组成部分，《中药炮制学》也已成为中药学类专业的必修课程。为使我国独具特色的炮制技术能够为世界所了解，亟需借助相应的载体，而《中药炮制学》双语教材将实现载体功能，有效地实现教学与传播的融合。这既能使中药学类专业的学生和广大中药行业从业人员在掌握中药炮制研究领域专业知识，了解和掌握相关的专业外语词汇，在具备从事中药炮制的教学、科研及开发应用能力的同时，相应提高英语水平，进一步增强其文化与技术沟通能力，又可帮助世界对中药炮制技术有所了解，为传承和发扬我国中医药事业奠定良好基础。

中药炮制学双语教材是以"十二五"国家级规划教材、全国高等中医药院校规划教材《中药炮制学》为依据编写完成。全书共12章，其中前5章分别介绍了中药炮制概述、炮制与临床疗效的关系、炮制目的、炮制辅料、炮制品质量要求与贮藏等，第6章至第12章则对炮制的具体过程，从净制、切制到具体炮制方法等，从品名、来源、炮制方法、炮制作用、炮制现代研究等方面对各饮片炮制进行论述。

参与本书编写的高等院校和研究院所包括辽宁中医药大学、上海中医药大学、天津中医药大学、南昌大学和山东科技大学。在编写过程中，山东科技大学的 David Karlau 和江西中医药大学的英文教师针对本书稿的英文文法进行了校正，同时得到了参与本书编写的院校和科研单位各级领导的热情鼓励和支持，在此一并表示深深的谢意！

由于编者水平有限，本书的不妥之处在所难免，请广大读者在使用本教材过程中提出宝贵意见，以便进一步修改提高。

《中药炮制学》双语教材编委会
2014 年 9 月

Written Description

Chinese materia medica processing (CMMP) is the exclusive pharmaceutical technology in China. The pieces of traditional Chinese drugs by processing, traditional Chinese medicine and Chinese patent drugs are called the three backbone of Chinese medicine industries. Discipline of CMMP based on TCM processing technology is the important composition in Chinese TCM disciplines. The course of CMMP has become the required discipline for TCM majors. In order to make this peculiar processing technology known by the world, corresponding vehicles are urgently needed. The bilingual textbook of CMMP can be one of the vehicles. It will be effective to realize the integration of teaching and spreading. Firstly, the students of TCM majors and general persons worked in TCM industry can grasp the knowledge of TCM processing, as well as understanding the professional English words . Meanwhile, people who had the ability of teaching, research, application in this field can also improve their English level and strengthen their communication ability of culture and technology. Secondly, with the help of this book, TCM processing can be achieved a good understanding by outside world. The publication of this book could provide a good foundation for inheriting and promoting of TCM throughout the world.

The bilingual textbook of *Processing of Chinese Materia Medica* is written based on "the 12th Five – Year Plan" National – level teaching materials and traditional Chinese Medicine Colleges teaching materials. It contains 12 chapters, in which the previous 5 chapters introduce the introduction, the relationship between processing and clinically therapeutic effectiveness, the purposes of processing, the supplemental material of CMMP and the quality control and storage of processed products. From the 6th chapter to 12th chapter, it elaborate the concrete procedure from purifying, cutting to the concrete CMMP skills, and expound the processing of each decoction pieces of traditional Chinese drugs which include the commodity name, source, processing method, processing function and modern research of drugs' processing.

The participating universities and research institutes to write the book include Liaoning University of TCM, Shanghai University of TCM, Tianjin University of TCM, Nanchang University and Shandong University of Science and Technology. In the process of compiling, David Karlau from Shandong University of Science and Technology and English teachers from Jiangxi University of TCM calibrate the manuscript grammar. We also get enthusiastic encourage and support of leaders from the partici-pating universities and research institutes. We give our deep gratitude to them.

For the limited of the editor, it will be unavoidable for some deficiency. Please put forward precious suggestion in the course of use for further improvement and modi-fication in the future.

Editorial Committee of Bilingual Textbook of CMMP

09 – 10 – 2014

Contents

目 录

Chapter One　Introduction

What is the meaning of the Chinese material medica processing (CMMP)? And what is the scientific principle of the Chinese material medica processing (CMMP)? When we get access to this ancient but young subject, we should broaden our vision to understand the function of the Chinese material medica processing (CMMP). At first, we should know the definition of the Chinese material medica processing (CMMP).

Section One　The Definition and Nature of Chinese Materia Medica Processing (CMMP)

1. The Definition of CMMP

According to the TCM theory, Chinese materia medica processing (CMMP) refers to a kind of pharmaceutical technology in accordance with the dialectical medication needs, the nature of the drugs itself, and the different requirements for compounding.

The broad sense: including cleansing, cutting and processing.

The narrow sense: including frying, stir – frying, calcining, steaming, boiling, blanching, repeated processing, fermentation, sprouting, frost – like powder making, baking, grinding in water, etc.

The definition of subject of CMMP: The science of CMMP is a subject specializing in the theory, technology, specification standard, history, and development.

About the theory of CMMP: It mainly refers to clarify the processing mechanism. Taking carbonizing drugs by stir – frying for example, the method can enhance its function of hematischesis. The TCM theory holds that "when red blood meets with black drugs, the former stops bleeding" (The five elements promotion and restriction mutually: metal – wood – water – fire – earth). While the modern theory believes that carbonizing drugs by stir – frying could increase the content of tannin, and promote blood clotting.

About the technology: The aim is to enhance the effect of processing and to standardize the processing technology. Taking Semen Strychni (*Maqianzi*) for example, there are stir – frying with sand technology, frying with oil technology, soaking in urine technology, and processing with vinegar technology. Among them, the soaking in urine technology is the distinctive processing method of Jiangxi Zhangbang. The aim of researching processing technology is to conserve the efficacy of medicines and improve the traditional technology.

About the specification standards: The aim is to standardize the types, specifications and quality standard of prepared drug in pieces, including cutting, thickness, vertical slices, transverse slices of the prepared drug in pieces, and the color standards of processed products, and to determine the quality standards of the processed products by applying modern research methods. Taking Semen Crotonis Pulveratum (*Badoushuang*) for example, the pharmacopoeia stipulates that the fatty oil in it should between 18% and 20%. Using the contents of strychnine as the indicator, the processing of Semen Strychni (*Maqianzi*) is included in the pharmacopoeia, thus standardizing and theorizing the processing and overcoming the limitations of the standards using experience to judge.

2. Basic Task of CMMP

Explore the principle of CMMP: The principle of CMMP refers to the scientific basis and the effect of CMMP, and the discussing of the physical change and chemical change of Chinese materia medica in the course of processing under certain technological conditions, and the pharmacological effects' changes originating from these changes, and the clinical significance owing to these changes, thus making certain scientific evaluation for processing methods. The principle covers such principle studies as reduction of side - effect, enhancement of efficacy, moderation of drug nature, generating of new efficacy, such as, the study of the processing mechanism of Radix Polygoni Multiflori (*Heshouwu*), Corydalis Rhizoma (*Yanhusuo*), etc.

Improve the technology of CMMP: The improvement of CMMP technology includes two aspects. First, improve the traditional processing technology. For example, Rhizoma Alismatis (*Zexie*) has been processed through the method of stir - frying with salt - water since the ancient times. But the modern research shows that, compared with the other processing technologies such as stir - frying Rhizoma Alismatis with bran, the efficacy of stir - frying Rhizoma Alismatis with salt - water makes no significant difference with them. We therefore believe that the method of stir - frying medicine with salt - water needs further discussion. Second, at present most of the prepared - drug - in - pieces transform the manual operation into the mechanical operation, which is the improvement of the CMMP technology, meanwhile promoting the large - scale production of prepared - drug - in - pieces industry.

Formulate quality standard of prepared drugs in pieces: In addition to experience of appearance differentiation, the quality standard of prepared drugs in pieces includes content of active ingredient, limitation of toxic ingredient, pesticide residue, heavy metals content, and research of fingerprinting similarity that has been discussed more in recent years.

3. Relationship between CMMP and Other Subjects

Relationship with the theory of TCM: The CMMP is the pharmaceutical technologies conducted under the direction of the T. C. M theory.

Relationship with chemistry of Chinese materia medica: To know about the principal constituents of drugs and their changes before and after processing, such as, Cortex Phellodendron contains berberine, which easily resolves in water. Therefore, when using water to process it, we should adopt the "as quickly as possible" means so as to avoid the loss of the effective constituents.

Relationship with analytical chemistry: Include two aspects, namely, chemical analysis and instrumental analysis. In chemical analysis, carrying on chemical analysis for raw and cooked products, judging which one is good and which one is bad through qualitative and quantitative analysis.

Relationship with identification of Chinese materia medica: Once the drugs are cut into small pieces, we could identify and distinguish the cross sections of prepared drugs in pieces through the knowledge of identification science.

Section Two   Origination and Development of CMMP

1. Origination of CMMP

The CMMP originated from the primitive society, developing along with the discovery of the Chinese materia medica. The CMMP is closely related with the invention of fire and the development of cooking skills (including the development of auxiliary materials and storage devices) .

2. Development of CMMP

The development of CMMP has gone through four stages, namely, the origination and formation period of CMMP technology, the formation period of processing theory, the expanding application period of processing varieties and technology, and the rejuvenation and development period of processing.

Section Three   Laws and Regulations of CMMP

Promulgated in December 2001, *the Drug Administration Law of the People' s Republic of China* (PRC) is the current basic law of drug production, use and inspection, and these are the laws and regulations that the Chinese materia medica processing must comply with.

In addition, the state – level laws and regulations include the *Pharmacopoeia of People's Republic of China*, whose appendix consists of the special chapter of the General Rules of the Chinese Materia Medica Processing (CMMP). The special chapter specifies the meaning of various processing methods, the operating methods sharing some general characteristics and quality requirements, being the state – level quality standards for traditional Chinese medicine processing.

Commissioned by the Bureau of Drug Administration of the Ministry of Public Health (Now National Health and Family Planning Commission of the People' s Republic of China) , the China Academy of T. C. M (Now China Academy of Chinese Medical Sciences) took the lead to organize the relevant units and personnel to compile the *National Specifications of Chinese Materia Medica Processing*, which was published in 1988, and has been adopted as the ministry – level processing standards of prepared Chinese drugs in pieces (tentative). The appendix contains the General Rules of the Chinese Materia Medica Processing (CMMP) and the National Profile of the Chinese Materia Medica Processing Methods, etc.

The local standards should be in line with the standards of state – level and ministry – level, under the circumstances that the varieties or projects are not included by the state – level and the ministry – level standards, can the local authorities formulate corresponding standards. Simultaneously, they should be reported to the drug supervision and management departments of the State Council for the record, such as, *Jiangxi Provincial Specifications of Chinese Materia Medica Processing*, *Fujian Provincial Specifications of Chinese Materia Medica Processing*, *Shaanxi Provincial Specifications of Chinese Materia Medica Processing*, etc.

第一章 概 述

中药炮制是什么？中药炮制的科学原理是什么？当接触这门古老而又年轻的学科时，我们应开阔视野去理解中药炮制的作用，首先需要了解的就是中药炮制的定义。

第一节 中药炮制的定义和性质

1. 中药炮制定义

根据中医药理论，按照辨证用药的需要和药物自身的性质及调剂制剂不同要求，所采取的一项制药技术，即为中药炮制。

广义：包括净制、切制和炮炙。

狭义：包括炒、炙、煅、蒸、煮、燀、复制、发酵、发芽、制霜、烘焙、水飞等。

中药炮制学定义：中药炮制学是专门研究中药炮制理论、工艺、规格标准、历史沿革及其发展的学科。

关于中药炮制理论：阐明炮制机理，例如药物炒炭后增强其止血作用，中医理论认为，"红见黑则止"（五行相生相克：金－木－水－火－土）。而现代理论则认为，药物炒炭后能增加鞣质含量，促进血凝。

关于工艺方面：目的在于提高炮制作用并规范炮制工艺。例如马钱子，有砂炒、油炸、尿泡、醋制，其中尿泡为江西樟帮的特色制法。炮制工艺研究的目的是保存药效的同时对传统工艺进行改进研究。

有关规格标准：目的在于规范饮片类型、规格和质量标准。包括饮片的切制、厚薄、纵片、横片，炮制品的色泽标准，以及应用现代研究确定炮制品的质量标准。如巴豆霜，药典规定其含脂肪油应为18%～20%；马钱子的炮制以士的宁含量作为指标载入药典，从而使炮制规范化、理论化，克服标准用经验判断的局限性。

2. 中药炮制学基本任务

探讨炮制原理：炮制原理是指药物炮制的科学依据和药物炮制的作用，即探讨在一定工艺条件下，中药在炮制过程中产生的物理变化和化学变化，以及因这些变化而产生的药理作用的改变和这些改变所产生的临床意义，从而对炮制方法作出一定的科学评价。它包括对降低副作用、增强疗效、缓和药性、产生新药效的原理研究等内容，例如对于何首乌、延胡索的炮制机理研究等。

　　改进炮制工艺：可从两方面来理解，首先是对传统炮制工艺的改进，如泽泻，从古至今都采用盐炙法进行炮制，但现代研究证明，盐炙泽泻的功效与其他炮制工艺，如麸炒泽泻等，并无明显区别，因此认为泽泻盐制还有待于进一步商榷。其次，目前大多数饮片厂都改手工操作为机械操作，也是对炮制工艺进行改进的一方面，可适应饮片工业的大生产需要。

　　制定饮片质量标准：饮片的质量标准包括经验外观鉴别，还需要增加对饮片的有效成分含量、有毒成分限量、农药残留量、重金属含量及目前讨论较多的指纹图谱相似度研究等。

3. 中药炮制学与其他学科关系

　　与传统中医药理论关系：中药炮制是在中医药理论指导下进行的制药技术。

　　与中药化学关系：了解药物的主要成分及炮制前后的变化，如黄柏中含有小檗碱，易溶于水，因此用水处理时，要采用"抢水洗"方式进行，避免有效成分的损失。

　　与分析化学关系：包括两方面，化学分析和仪器分析。在化学分析方面，对药物的生熟制品进行化学分析，通过定性定量来判断孰优孰劣。

　　与中药鉴定的关系：药物切制成饮片之后可通过鉴定学知识的掌握对饮片断面进行鉴定判别。

第二节　中药炮制的起源和发展

1. 中药炮制的起源

　　中药炮制起源于原始社会，随着中药的发现而发展，并与火的发明、烹饪技术的发展密切相关（包括辅料和贮存器的发展）。

2. 中药炮制的发展

　　中药炮制发展经历了四个阶段：中药炮制技术的起始和形成时期；炮制理论的形成时期；炮制品种和技术的扩大应用时期；炮制振兴和发展时期。

第三节　中药炮制的法规

　　2001 年 12 月颁布的《中华人民共和国药品管理法》，是目前药品生产、使用、检验的基本法律，这便是中药炮制所必须遵守的法规。

　　此外国家级法规包括《中华人民共和国药典》，附录设有"中药炮制通则"专篇，规定了各种炮制方法的含义、具有共性的操作方法及质量要求，是属国家级中药炮制的质量标准。

　　《全国中药炮制规范》由卫生部（现卫生和计划生育委员会）药政局委托中国中医研

究院（现中国中医科学院）牵头组织有关单位及人员编写而成，于1988年出版，作为部级中药饮片炮制标准（暂行），附录中收录了"中药炮制通则"及"全国中药炮制法概况表"等。

　　地方标准应与国家、部颁标准一致，在国家与部级标准没有收载相应品种或项目的情况下，可制定相应的地方标准，同时应当报国务院药品监督管理部门备案，如《江西省中药炮制规范》《福建省中药炮制规范》《陕西省中药炮制规范》等。

Chapter Two　The Chinese Materia Medica Processing and Clinical Efficacy

Section One　The Relationship between CMMP and Clinical Efficacy

The Chinese Materia Medica Processing (CMMP) is the medication features of Chinese Medicine. First, prepared Chinese drugs in pieces are the material foundation of the TCM clinical medication. Second, the theory of Chinese medicine is the guidance of the CMMP. Third, it can change drugs' effects through CMMP to meet the clinical needs is the fundamental guarantee for TCM clinical medication.

According to TCM theories, the clinical of Chinese medicine is closely related to cleansing, cutting, heating and adjuvant materials.

Suitable cleansing procedure could remove impurities and non – medicinal parts of drugs, a-voiding mixing other drugs, and eliminating toxicity of some drugs.

Cutting can affect the clinical efficacy through changing thickness and size of drugs. At the same time, suitable drying temperature and time are critical in affecting the quality of prepared drugs in pieces.

Heating can be divided into two types, namely, dry heating and humid heating. The former includes the processing methods such as simple stir – frying, fried with solid adjuvant materials, calcining and so on, which can make drugs' texture crisper and easy to decoct effective sub-stances. The latter includes stir – frying, steaming, boiling, etc. , which make drugs more suitable for clinical needs. For example, stir – frying Radix Angelicae Sinensis (*Danggui*) with wine pro-motes blood circulation for removing blood stasis, replenishing blood and regulating menstruation.

The adjuvant materials of processing could be divided into two categories, namely, the solid and liquid adjuvant materials. The solid adjuvant materials include rice, soil, sand, etc. , which can conduct heat and make drugs heat evenly. The liquid adjuvant materials include wine, vine-gar, honey, etc. , which permeate into the interior of drugs and change physical and chemical properties of drugs. For example, after being stir – fried with wine, the effect of Rhizoma Coptidis (*Huanglian*) would be elevated to clear away upper – energizer damp – heat of a body. After being stir – fried with vinegar, the effect of Rhizoma Corydalis (*Yanhusuo*) would be conducted to reach liver channels to soothe liver and disperse stagnant liver *qi*. After being stir – fried with salt water, the effect of Cortex Phellodendri Chinensis (*Huangbo*) would be conducted to reach kidney channels to nourish *yin* and purge fire. After being stir – fried with ginger juice, Cortex Magnoliae Officinalis (*Houpo*) would have dispersing function and have more effect on reliving epigastric distension and removing stagnation. After being stir – fried with honey, the Flos Farfarae (*Kuandonghua*) would become sweet and have more effect on relieving cough and replenishing *qi*.

Section Two   The Traditional Pharmaceutical Principles

In the Qing Dynasty, Xu Lingtai summed the traditional pharmaceutical principles as the following aspects: processing on clashing, processing on assistance, processing on restraint, and processing on inhibition. The concrete methods include processing for shape, processing for property, processing for flavor, and processing for texture.

Processing on clashing: It refers to the method of processing drugs with adjuvant materials (including drugs) whose property is opposite to that of processed drugs. The purpose is to restrain drugs' side effects or to alter their properties. For example, processing bitter, cold and sinking – descending properties of Radix et Rhizoma Rhei (*Dahuang*) with pungent, hot and ascending – lifting properties wine, could transfer its descending property to ascending property.

Processing on assistance: It refers to using the method of processing drugs with adjuvant materials whose property is similar to that of processed drugs to enhance drugs' efficacy. For example, processing bitter cold property of Rhizoma Anemarrhenae (*Zhimu*) and Cortex Phellodendri Chinensis (*Huangbo*) with cold salt solution could increase the effects of nourishing *yin* to purge fire. Processing Radix Glycyrrhizae (*Gancao*) with honey could increase its effects of invigorating spleen – stomach and replenishing *qi*.

Processing on restraint: It refers to processing drugs by using some adjuvant materials to reduce toxicity or side – effects. For example, Rhizoma Zingiberis Recens (*Shengjiang*) can detoxify the toxin of Rhizoma Pinelliae (*Banxia*) and Rhizoma Arisaematis (*Tiannanxing*), so using Rhizoma Zingiberis Recens (*Shengjiang*) to process Rhizoma Pinelliae (*Banxia*) and Rhizoma Arisaematis (*Tiannanxing*).

Processing on mutual inhibition: It refers to processing drugs with some adjuvant materials (or drugs) to moderate drastic property to prevent vital *qi* from being damaged. For example, stir – frying Rhizoma Atractylodis Macrocephalae (*Baizhu*) with bran can moderate its dryness nature.

Processing for form: It refers to changing drugs' outward forms and separating its different medicinal parts by processing.

Processing for property: It refers to changing drugs' properties by processing. The properties include cold, hot, warm and cool property and actions of ascending, descending, floating and sinking.

Processing for flavor: It refers to regulating drugs' five flavors including pungent, sweet, sour, bitter and salty, or rectifying their bad flavors.

Processing for texture: It refers to changing drugs' properties or textures by processing.

Section Three　The Influence of Processing on Drugs' Properties

1. The Influence of Processing on Four Natures and Five Flavors

The influence of processing on drugs' natures and flavors is as follows.

The first aspect is to strengthen drugs' original natures and flavors by processing with adjuvant materials or drugs whose properties are similar to the processed drugs, which is called adjuvant processing. When it is processed with cold and bitter bile, the cold and bitter property of Rhizoma Coptidis (*Huanglian*) will be strengthened, which is called making the cold colder. When Rhizoma Curculigins (*Xianmao*) is processed with pungent and hot wine, its effect of warming kidneys to invigorate *yang* will be strengthened, which is called making the hot hotter.

The second aspect is to rectify drugs' side – effects by processing with adjuvant materials or drugs whose properties are opposite to the processed drugs, which is called inhibitory processing. When the cold and bitter Rhizoma Coptidis (*Huanglian*) is processed with pungent and warm ginger juice, its cold and bitter property will be moderated, which is called inhibiting the cold by the hot.

The third aspect is to widen drugs' application due to altering drugs' natures and flavors by processing. Radix Rehmanniae Recens (*Shengdi*) is cold in nature and sweet in taste, with the effects of clearing heat and cooling blood, nourishing *yin* and promoting production of body fluid. However, Radix Rehmanniae Praeparata (*Shudihuang*) turns into one with warm and sweet properties, with the effects of nourishing *yin* and tonifying blood. So the unprocessed one is cold in nature with the main effect of clearing – away pathogenic fire, while the prepared one is warm in nature with the main effect of tonifying blood. Rhizoma Arisaematis (*Tiannanxing*) is pungent and warm with the effects of drying dampness and resolving phlegm, and dispelling wind for resolving convulsion. But when it is processed with bile, it turns into cool and bitter in nature, and has the effects of clearing heat and dissipating phlegm, and extinguish wind and arresting convulsion.

2. The Influence of Processing on the Actions of Ascending, Descending, Floating and Sinking

Actions of ascending, descending, floating and sinking refer to the tendency of drugs' acting on body, which are closely related to drugs' natures and flavors. The drug's acting tendency may be altered due to its change of nature and flavor after it is processed. For example, Cortex Phellodendri Chinensis (*Huangbo*) has the effect of clearing – away dampness – heat in the lower energizer originally. It can also clear away damp – heat in the upper energizer after it is processed with wine. Semen Raphani (*Laifuzi*) has the actions of both ascending and descending. The raw one mainly ascends with the effect of causing emetic of the wind – phlegm, while the stir – fried one mainly descends with the effects of directing *qi* downward and resolving phlegm, promoting digestion and removing food stagnation.

3. The Influence of Processing on Channel Tropism

Channel tropism refers to drugs' selective effect on a certain part of body. Drugs may exert obvious or specific effect on the pathological changes in one or several certain viscera and meridian, and with small effect on the others. After drugs are processed, the channel tropism, which the drugs mainly act on, may be changed. The drugs' effect may more focus on one or some certain viscera or meridian, but less on the others. For example, Rhizoma Anemarrhenae (*Zhimu*) acts on lungs, stomachs and kidneys, with the effects of clearing away heat from lungs, stomachs and removing ministerial fire. But after stir – frying with salt – water, it mainly acts on kidneys with the effect of nourishing *yin* for lowering fire.

4. The Influence of Processing on Toxicity

The purpose of removing drugs' toxicity may be obtained by processing. And the frequently – used methods are cleansing, soaking and rinsing with water, grinding in water, processing with adjuvant materials, and frosting by defatting, etc.

第二章　中药炮制与临床疗效

第一节　中药炮制与临床疗效的关系

中药炮制是中医用药的特点，一是因为中药饮片是中医临床用药的物质基础，二是中药炮制必须在中医药理论指导下进行，三是通过中药炮制可改变药效以适应临床需要，是中医临床用药的根本保证。

中医药理论认为，中医临床与炮制的净制、切制、加热制和辅料制密切相关。

通过净制可以去除药物中的杂质和非药用部位，防止混药并去除某些药物的毒性。

切制可以通过改变饮片的厚薄和大小来影响临床疗效，与此同时，适宜的干燥温度和时间对饮片质量的影响也至关重要。

加热可以分为干热和湿热两种，其中干热炮制包括清炒、加固体辅料炒、煅等，可使药物质地酥脆，易于煎出药效物质。湿热炮制包括炙、蒸、煮等，可使药物更适合临床需求。例如，酒炙当归，可增强活血化瘀、补血调经的功效。

炮制辅料可分为两类，即固体辅料和液体辅料。固体辅料包括米、土、砂等，具有传热和使药物受热均匀的作用。液体辅料包括酒、醋、蜜等，可渗入到药材内部并使之发生理化改变。例如，黄连经酒炙后，可引药上行，清上焦湿热；延胡索经醋炙后，可引药入肝，舒肝解郁；黄柏经盐炙后，可引药入肾，滋阴降火；厚朴经姜炙后，具有发散作用，并增强宽中散满功效；款冬花经蜜炙后，味甘并增强止咳和益气作用。

第二节　传统的制药原则

清代徐灵胎将传统的制药原则归纳为：相反为制，相资为制，相畏为制，相恶为制。具体方法为：或制其形，或制其性，或制其味，或制其质。

相反为制：是指用药性相对立的辅料（包括药物）来制约中药的偏性或改变药性。如用辛热升提的酒来炮制苦寒沉降的大黄，使药性转降为升。

相资为制：是指用药性相似的辅料或某种炮制方法来增强药效。如用咸寒的盐水炮制苦寒的知母、黄柏，可增强滋阴降火作用。蜜炙甘草可增强补中益气作用。

相畏（或相杀）为制：是指利用某种辅料来炮制药物，以制约该药物的毒副作用。如生姜能杀半夏、南星毒（即半夏、南星畏生姜），故用生姜来炮制半夏、南星。

相恶为制： 是指用某种辅料（或药物）或某种方法来减弱药物的烈性，以免损伤正气。如麸炒白术可使其燥性得到缓和。

制其形： 是指改变药物的外观形态和分开药用部位。

制其性： 是指通过炮制改变药物的性能，如寒、热、温、凉或升、降、浮、沉的性质。

制其味： 是指通过炮制，调整中药的五味（如辛、甘、酸、苦、咸）或矫正劣味。

制其质： 即通过炮制改变药物的性质或质地。

第三节　炮制对药性的影响

1. 炮制对四气五味的影响

炮制对性味的影响大致有三种情况：

一是用药性相似的辅料或药物进行炮制，使药物的性味增强，又称为"从制"。如以苦寒的胆汁制黄连，更增强了黄连的苦寒之性，所谓寒者益寒；以辛热的酒制仙茅，增强了仙茅的温肾壮阳作用，所谓热者益热。

二是用药性相反的辅料或药物进行炮制，以纠正药物过偏之性，又称为"反制"。如黄连苦寒之性甚强，经过辛温的姜汁制后，能降低苦寒之性，即所谓以热制寒。

三是通过炮制，改变药物性味，扩大药物的用途。如生地甘寒，具有清热凉血、养阴生津作用；制成熟地后，则转为甘温之品，具有滋阴补血的功效。即一者性寒，主清；一者性温，主补。天南星辛温，善于燥湿化痰、祛风止痉；加胆汁制成胆南星，则性味转为苦凉，具有清热化痰、息风定惊的功效。

2. 炮制对升降浮沉的影响

升降浮沉是指药物作用于机体的趋向，与中药的性味关系密切。药物经炮制后，由于性味的变化，可以改变其作用趋向。如黄柏原系清下焦湿热之药，经酒制后作用向上，能清上焦之热。莱菔子能升能降，生品以升为主，用于涌吐风痰；炒后则以降为主，长于降气化痰，消食除胀。

3. 炮制对归经的影响

归经就是指药物对机体某部位的选择性作用，药物可能对某些脏腑或经络表现出明显的作用，而对其他脏腑或经络的作用不明显或无作用。药物经炮制后，作用重点可以发生变化，其中某一脏腑或经络的作用增强，而对其他脏腑或经络的作用相应地减弱，使其功效更加专一。如知母入肺、胃、肾经，具有清肺、凉胃、泻相火的作用，盐炙后则主要作用于肾经，可增强滋阴降火的功效。

4. 炮制对药物毒性的影响

药物通过炮制，可以达到去毒的目的。去毒常用的炮制方法有净制、水泡漂、水飞、加辅料处理、去油制霜等。

Chapter Three   The Purposes of Processing and Its Influences on Drugs

Section One   The Purposes of Processing

Chinese materia medica comes from plants, animals and minerals, some of which are hard and thick in texture, some of which contain impurities and sands, and some of which have larger side effects. Generally they cannot be directly used in clinical practise, they must be processed into prepared Chinese drugs in pieces before they are used for clinical purposes. The purposes of processing are various. A drug may have multiple effects owing to different processing methods. Though these effects could be differentiated as primary and secondary, they are also closely related to each other. The purposes of processing are mentioned below.

1. Reducing or Removing Toxicity or Side - effects of Drugs

Some drugs with apparent efficacy maybe not so safe on clinical application for their strong toxicity or side – effects. But the toxicity and side – effects can be reduced by processing. For example, the toxicity and side – effects of Radix Aconiti Kusnezoffii (*Caowu*) can be reduced by soaking, rinsing with water, steaming, boiling and processing with adjuvant materials. Similarly, the toxicity of Radix Phytolaccae (*Shanglu*) and Fructus Xanthii (*Cang'erzi*) could be reduced after processing.

Processing can also remove or reduce drugs' side – effects. It is said that the raw Herba Ephedrae (*Mahuang*) induces fidgety and continuous sweating according to *Jinguiyuhanjing* by Zhang Zhongjing, a famous medical expert in the Han dynasty. Boiling it several times may reduce its side – effects. Another example, when meeting with cases with insomnia, uneasiness and loose stools, we should use Semen Platycladi (*Baiziren*) to nourish hearts and tranquilize mind. But Semen Platycladi (*Baiziren*) have the side – effects of moistening intestine and inducing diarrhea, after taking it, diarrhea would occur. The side – effects can be avoided by frosting and by defatting.

2. Altering or Alleviating Drugs' Properties

Chinese materia medica is described as cold, hot, warm, cool (namely "four properties") in nature; and pungent, sweet, sour, bitter and salty (namely "five flavors") in flavor. The drugs with drastic properties and flavors may have some side – effects. Too much coldness damages *yang*, too much hotness damages *yin*, super pungency consumes body fluid and *qi*, super sweet induces dampness, peracid damages teeth, super bitterness damages stomach, and super saltiness induces phlegm. Drugs' nature and flavors can be altered or alleviated by processing. Sun Simiao, a famous medical expert in the Tang dynasty, ever said that Ramulus Cinnamomi (*Guizhi*) should be boiled when it is used for pregnant women to prevent fetal movement. Luo Zhouyan in the Ming dynasty, said "Fructus Aurantii (*Zhiqiao*) which could promote digestion and relieve dyspepsia should be stir – fried with bran, or it could damage original *qi*". The raw Herba Ephedrae (*Mahuang*) is strong in the effects of expelling exogenous evils from body surfaces with its pungent flavor. And if it is processed with honey, its volatile oil content with the effect of relieving exterior syndrome with pungent warm and cool nature decreases, and then the above effects will be moderated. Refined honey has the nature of moisturizing dryness and has synergistic effect with Herba Ephedrae (*Mahuang*), and the effect of relieving cough and asthma will be increased. The later generations have often used the processing methods like stir – frying or stir – frying with honey to moderate drugs' properties, and have summarized the rules that sweet can moderate drugs' properties, and stir – frying can alleviate drugs' properties.

After being processed, drugs could change their original properties, producing different clinical efficacies. For example, raw Pollen Typhae (*Puhuang*) can promote blood circulation to remove blood stasis, while the stir – fried one can stop bleeding. Raw Radix Glycyrrhizae (*Gancao*) with sweet taste and cool property can clear away heat and relieve toxicity, but after being processed with honey, its property transfers to sweet and warm, being good at invigorating spleen and replenishing *qi*, relieving spasm and pain. So when the drugs are used for tonifying, it should be processed with honey, while the unprocessed drugs are used as cathartic.

3. Strengthening Drugs' Efficacy

In addition to the combination with other drugs, processing is another effective means to strengthen drugs' efficacy. The proper processing methods can increase dissolution rates of active ingredients of drugs and make the extractives be absorbed easily so as to strengthen efficacy. The ancients believed that "All the seed drugs like Catsia tora Linn (*Juemingzi*), Semen Raphani (*Laifuzi*), Semen Sinapis Albae (*Baijiezi*), Fructus Perillae (*Zisuzi*), Semen Allii Tuberosi (*Jiucaizi*) and Semen Celosiae (*Qingxiangzi*) must be stir – fried so as to make their flavors come out". Because it is difficult to extract seeds' active ingredients from its hard shells. But frying seeds can make extraction easy by bursting seeds. That's why almost all seeds and fruits need to be stir – fried. Meanwhile, the effects of nourishing lungs for arresting cough of some expectorants and antitussive drugs, such as Flos Farfarae (*Kuandonghua*), Radix Asteris (*Ziwan*), are increased after being processed with honey. Refined honey has the efficacy of tonifying spleen with mild sweet nature and moistening lung for arresting cough. When it is used as adjuvant material, it could work co – operatively with drugs, thus enhancing the efficacy. The modern experiments have showed that the effect of relieving spasm of Rhizoma Arisaematis (*Tiannanxing*) is increased after it is processed with bile. The bacteriostasis of Rhizoma Coptidis (*Huanglian*) is increased by several times after it is processed with decoction of Radix Glycyrrhizae (*Gancao*). Obviously, after being processed, the drugs efficacy could be enhanced from different aspects.

4. Altering or Strengthening Drugs' Acting Location and Tendency

According to the theory of TCM, the location, on which a drug acts, is expressed by meridian and viscera, and the tendency of drugs' actions is expressed by ascending, descending, sinking and floating. Chinese materia medica could change their effect tends through processing. Meanwhile, pathogenesis and syndromes of diseases also have the ascending and descending properties. For example, cough, asthma, hemoptysis, etc. , present the ascending properties. While diarrhea, hemorrhage uterine, enuresis present the descending properties. These functional disturbances of organisms can be corrected by the drugs' acting tendency. Processing can lead the drugs to target a certain meridian and alter the drugs' acting locations and tendency. For example, Radix et Rhizoma Rhei (*Dahuang*) is bitter in taste, cold in nature, and sinking in action. Processing it with wine may guide it to the upper – energizer. Cortex Phellodendri (*Huangbai*), supreme *yin* in nature, tasteless in smell, greasy in flavor, and descending in tendency, when processing it with wine, the properties may transfer from descending to ascending, and clear fire of the upper – energizer.

Clinically, if a drug reaches several meridians, its effects would be dispersed. Processing can make it focus on one certain part. For example, Radix Bupleuri (*Chaihu*), which is attributive to the meridians of liver, gallbladder and triple – energizer. Its effects concentrate on the liver meridian and shows stronger effectiveness after being processed. Our predecessors summed up some laws about this, such as "The raw is ascending while the processed is descending" "Processing with wine makes drugs' properties ascending and floating" and "Processing with salt water leads it to the kidney meridian", etc.

5. Facilitating Prescription and Preparation

After being processed by water to become soft and cut into pieces, filaments, sections and lumps with certain specifications, Chinese herbal medicine coming from the plant class, such as root, stems, rattan, wood, flower, leaf and grass could be advantageous for dividing doses and filling prescriptions when dispensing. Minerals, shells and animal bones, such as Pyritum (*Zirantong*), Squama Manis (*Chuanshanjia*), Tortoise Plastron (*Guiban*), Turtle Shells (*Biejia*), Semen Strychni (*Maqianzi*), Asini Corii Colla (*E'jiao*), are difficult to be crushed due to their hard texture. They must be processed by calcining, quenching or stir – frying with sand or Pulvis Talci (*Huashifen*), which can make their texture crisp and easy to be crushed so that the active ingredients could be easily extracted, and absorbed by human bodies.

6. Facilitating Storage and Keeping Effectiveness

Drying drugs to decrease its moisture content avoids rotting and deteriorating, and makes them easy to be stored. Boiling, steaming and stir – frying insect and animal class drugs like Oötheca Mantidis (*Sangpiaoxiao*) could kill ova in the drugs to avoid incubation. At the same time, processing seeds by steaming, stir – frying and scalding can avoid germination. Heating the drugs containing glycoside such as Radix Scutellariae (*Huangqin*), Semen Armeniacae Amarum (*Kuxingren*) that destroy the active properties of the enzyme to avoid the loss of active glycoside and the reducing of efficacy.

7. Rectifying Drugs' Fishy Smells and Terrible Odors

Some animal drugs (such as Placenta Hominis – *Ziheche*, Endoconcha Sepiae – *Haipiaoxiao*), the resinous herbs (such as Resina Olibani – *Ruxiang*, Resina Myrrhae – *Moyao*), or other drugs with terrible odors are hard to be taken orally or result in side – effects, such as nausea, emesis and vexation. To facilitate administration of these drugs, the processing methods such as processing with wine or honey, rinsing, stir – frying with bran, stir – bake to yellow should be taken to rectify the bad odors, such as, processing Zaocys (*Wushaoshe*) with wine, and stir – frying Bombyx Batryticatus (*Jiangcan*) with bran.

8. Making Drugs Pure to Ensure Quality

Drugs are often mixed up with sand, impurities, residual non – medicinal parts and rotten products during collecting, storing, and transporting. Before they are used in clinical practice, they must be strictly processed by separating, cleaning and washing to ensure health and exact dosage. For example, rhizome of root class drugs (rhizome parts of upper roots), coarse skins in bark drugs (cork bark), and heads, feet and wings of insect drugs should be removed. The different medicinal parts sometimes also should be separated for clinical applications although they are from the same plants. For example, stem of Herba Ephedrae (*Mahuang*) can induce sweating while its roots can stop sweating, so they must be used separately to meet the different medical demands.

Section Two　The Influence of Processing on Drugs' Chemical Composition

The chemical composition of a drug is the basis of its clinical effect. The chemical compositions of Chinese materia medica are rather complicated, and people are unclear about the condition of some effective ingredients. The functions of Chinese materia medica are comprehensive, some of which are cooperative and some are antagonistic. A series of changes on chemical compositions take place after drugs are heated, soaked with water and processed with wine, vinegar or the decoction of other drugs. Some compositions' contents increase while some others decrease or disappear, or some new compounds come into being. So it is important to study the changes of chemical compositions after processing, and it is the basis for discussing the processing action and mechanism of

Chinese materia medica. But because the effective ingredients of most Chinese materia medica are not clear and the time of researching on this aspect is short, with less accumulated data, until now, we can't expound the influence of processing on the chemical compositions of drugs entirely and profoundly. The influence of processing on the main effective ingredients can be described as below.

1. The Influence of Processing on Drugs Containing Alkaloid

Alkaloid is an organic compound containing nitrogen with alkaline property. Many of them are bitter in taste and have apparent biological activity. Not only plant drugs but also some animal drugs such as Venenum Bufonis (*Chansu*) contain alkaloid.

A free alkaloid slightly dissolves in water, but easily dissolves in ethanol, chloroform and other organic solvents, and it can also dissolve in acid solution. Most alkaloid salts dissolve in water, but can't or hardly dissolve in organic solvents, so wine and vinegar, etc., are often used as adjuvant materials to process drugs containing alkaloid to improve dissolution rate of alkaloid.

Wine is considered as both polar solvent and non - polar solvent, a good solvent. Alcohol is often used to extract the ingredients of Chinese materia medica, and wine is a kind of liquid adjuvant material having the nature of diluting alcohol. Whether free alkaloids or their alkaloid salts can dissolve in wine easily. The extracting rate of alkaloids and the drugs' efficacy increase after it is processed with wine.

Vinegar is a kind of weak acid and it can combine free alkaloids to form salt. Alkaloid acetate dissolves in water easily, which increases the content of active ingredients in the water solution and improves drugs' efficacy. For example, the main effective ingredients of Rhizoma Corydalis (*Yanhusuo*) are tetrahydropalmatine and dehydrocorydaline, having the effects of analgesia and sedation. These two alkaloids exist in the medicinal materials in the form of free alkaloids, hard to dissolve in water. But after being processed with vinegar, these alkaloids can conjugate with acetic acid to form alkaloid acetate, which is easy to dissolve in water. So after processing Rhizoma Corydalis (*Yanhusuo*) with vinegar, the analgesic effect will be enchanced.

Alkaloids often form compound salts with organic acid and inorganic acid in plants, such as tannate and oxalate, which are difficult to dissolve in water. Acetic acid can replace the acids mentioned above and form acetate salt, which increases their solubility in water.

Most alkaloids can't dissolve in water, but some small molecule alkaloids, such as arecoline, and some quaternary ammonium compounds, such as berberine, dissolve in water. When the drugs containing such alkaloids are washed or soaked in water, we should minimize the time that alkaloids contact with water. We should remember the principle of "little soaking but much moistening" when cutting them, and we should, as much as possible, reduce the loss of alkaloids during the course of soaking so as not to affect the efficacy.

Different alkaloids have different heat resistances. Some alkaloids aren't stable in the condition of high temperature, causing hydrolysis and decomposition. The structures of alkaloids can be changed by such processing methods as boiling, steaming, frying, scalding, calcining or stir -

frying, etc. , so as to reduce the toxicity and strengthen the effect. For example, in the condition of high temperature, aconitine can be hydrolyzed into aconitum alkali and aconine, which is much less toxic than aconitine. So processing can guarantee the safety and effectiveness in clinical applications. The alkaloids in such drugs as Radix Sophorae Tonkinensis (*Shandougen*) are effective substances, whose activity will decrease when being heated, so we'd better reduce the process of heat treatment and use the raw ones.

2. The Influence of Processing on Drugs Containing Glycoside

The glycosides are widely distributed in nature, existing in many parts of plants, especially in fruits, barks and roots.

The dissolubility of glycoside doesn' t have apparent regularity. Generally they dissolve in water or ethanol, and some of them dissolve in chloroform and ethylacetate, but they are hard to dissolve in ether and benzene. The number of sugar molecules and the polar group on aglucon also influence the solubility. The more the number of the polar groups on aglycone, the higher the solubility in water. Otherwise, the solubility in water is lower.

As a commonly used adjuvant material in processing, wine can increase the solubility of drugs containing glycoside, which can strengthen the efficacy. Because glycoside dissolves in water easily, we should also adopt the principle of "little soaking but much moistening" when processing such drugs with water in order to avoid the loss of glycoside, or the decrease owing to hydrolysis. Such drugs include Radix et Rhizoma Rhei (*Dahuang*), Radix Glycyrrhizae (*Gancao*), Cortex Fraxini (*Qinpi*), etc. They all contain many kinds of glycoside dissolving in water, and need extreme caution when treating with water before cutting.

The drugs containing glycoside often contain relevant decomposing enzymes. The glycoside can be hydrolyzed by the enzyme under proper temperatures and humidity, which can decrease the content of active glycoside and weaken the drugs' efficacy. Meanwhile, after being collected and stored for long time, the relevant enzymes in some drugs, for example Flos Sophorae (*Huaihua*), Semen Armeniacae Amarum (*Kuxingren*) and Radix Scutellariae (*Huangqin*) may decompose active rutin, amygdalin and baicalin respectively, which weaken the drugs' effectiveness. Sometimes, anthocyanin in flowers also changes color and loses petals due to the effect of enzymes. So we often process such drugs by frying, steaming, baking, scalding or insolating to destroy or inhibit the activity of enzyme to protect the glycoside from hydrolyzing, preserving the drug efficacy.

Glycoside is easy to be hydrolyzed in acid conditions, which not only decreases glycoside' s contents but also increases the complexity of the ingredients. So if glycoside is the effective ingredient of drugs, it should be avoided to be processed with vinegar or occasionally with vinegar except specialized medical requirements.

3. The Influence of Processing on Drugs Containing Volatile Oil

Volatile oil is a kind of ingredient having efficacy, and it also known as essential oil. Under normal temperature, it is a kind of free running oil – like liquid. Volatile oil has fragrance and volatility, and generally refers to the generic name of volatile oil – like ingredient obtained through steam distillation. Volatile oil generally has fragrance. It can volatilize voluntarily at normal temperature without leaving any oil stains. Most of them are lighter than water, and they can dissolve in many organic solvents and fatty oils easily. They can completely dissolve in 70%, or higher concentration ethanol. The volatile oil has low solubility in water.

Long time ago, people have already known there were aromatic volatile ingredients in many plants. They indicated that these drugs should be given minimum heating or should not be heated. For example, in *Lei's Treatise on Preparation of Drugs* (*Leigongpaozhilun*), it was said that Herba Artemisiae Scopariae (*Yinchen*) shouldn't be heated by fire. In *Compendium of Materia Medica* (*Bencaogangmu*), it was recorded that Radix Aucklandiae (*Muxiang*) shouldn't be heated with fire when it is used for promoting *qi*, but when it is used to nourish large intestines, it should be roasted in fresh cinders covered with flour. So the crude drugs containing volatile oil should be promptly treated and dried in shade. They should be washed quickly to avoid loss of volatile oil. More attention should be paid when they need to be heated.

Some volatile oil of drugs should be reduced or removed by processing to meet the clinical needs. For example, Herba Ephedrae (*Mahuang*) should be processed with honey to reduce the content of volatile oil with the function of inducing sweat by 50%, while the content of ephedrine with the function of relieving dyspnea basically is not affected. Combined with honey's complementary role, honey – stirred Herba Ephedrae (*Mahuang*) is more suitable for treatment of asthma. Another example, Rhizoma Atractylodi (*Cangzhu*) contains much volatile oil, which is thought as irritant and drastic according to the theory of TCM. The experimental results showed that the content of volatile oil in Rhizoma Atractylodi (*Cangzhu*) can be reduced by 80% by stir – frying the drug to charcoal, reduced by 40% by stir – frying it to brown, reduced by 20% by roasting or stir – frying it with earth, and reduced by 10% to 15% by processing it with vinegar, wine, salt – water, rice – washed water and stir – frying with bran. Different processing methods should be adopted according to different clinical demands.

Drug processing not only alters the volatile content, but also causes qualitative changes. For example, the color becomes darker, refractive index increases, some new components are produced and pharmacological effect alters. It is said that nine new kinds of crud schizonepeta oil are found in Herba Schizonepetae Carbonisata (*Jingjietan*) which could be used for stopping bleeding. After being roasted, Semen Myristicae's (*Roudoukou*) function of inhibiting isolated intestinal contraction in rabbits is strengthened, resulting in antidiarrheal effect. The volatile oil of some drugs has apparent toxicity and strong irritation, the majority of which can be removed by processing, which is conducive to clinical application. For example, volatile oil of Resina Olibani (*Ruxiang*) has strong stomach irritation and causes vomiting, the crude drug is often for external use. Most volatile oil can be removed after processed, and its toxicity and irritation is reduced, available for oral administration. Thus, the volatile oil in certain raw medicinal material has the obvious toxicity and very strong irritating quality, we can meet the clinical requirements by processing them.

Most volatile oils in plants exist in free state, and some of them exist in combining state. For Herba Menthae (*Bohe*) and Herba Schizonepetae (*Jingjie*) existing in free state, we should rapidly process and cut them after collecting or spraying. They should not be stacked with water for long time to avoid being fermented and affect quality. But for other plants, the volatile oils exist in combining state, which should be piled up to ferment to free the fragrance. For example, Cortex Magnoliae Officinalis (*Houpo*), should be buried to ferment to produce high quality prepared herbal medicine.

4. The Influence of Processing on Drugs Containing Tannins

Tannin, a kind of complicated compound of phenols with certain physiological activities, exists widely in plants. It is often used as an astringent for stopping bleeding, relieving diarrhea, antibiosis, and defending mucosa, etc. It can also be used as an antidote for poisoning of alkaloids and heavy metals.

Tannin dissolves in water easily, especially in hot water. It involves many phenolic hydroxyls so it has strong polarity. When being treated with water, the drugs containing tannin as the main active ingredient such as Radix Sanguisorbae (*Diyu*) should be paid much attention.

Tannin is a kind of strong reducing agent and can be oxidized by the oxygen in the air to become red. This is the reason why Semen Arecae (*Binglang*) and Radix Paeoniae Alba (*Baishao*) become red once they are exposed in air for a long time. The color of tannin changes more rapidly in alkaline solvent, which must be paid special attention to when being processed.

Tannin is thermally stable, so it doesn't change a lot when it is heated at a high temperature. For example, Radix et Rhizoma Rhei (*Dahuang*) contains anthraquinone glycoside with the action of diarrhea and tannin with the astringent function. When it is steamed with wine and is carbonized by stir – frying, the content of anthraquinone glycoside decreases significantly, but the content of tannin remains basically unchanged, so relatively the purgative function is reduced, and the astringent function is strengthened. If the decocting time is too long, the anthraquinone glycoside is destroyed completely, so the drugs would no longer to purge but induce constipation. In some condition, tannin's efficacy may be affected by processing at a high temperature. For example, when Radix Sanguisorbae (*Diyu*) is carbonized at too high temperature, its bacteriostasis action would be weakened largely. For such drugs, we should control the heating time and heating temperature when processing.

Chemical reactions will happen when tannin meets iron. Tannin will be transferred to tannin molysite precipitation of black – green. So, in order to avoid reacting with iron, when cutting drugs containing tannin, we should use bamboo knives or steel knives. When washing, the drugs containing tannin should be placed in wood basins. When decocting, the drugs containing tannin should be put in a marmite instead of an iron pan.

5. The Influence of Processing on Drugs Containing Organic Acid

Organic acid widely exists in the cell juice of plants, especially in immature pulpy fruits. The contents of organic acid decrease gradually along with the fruits maturing. The common organic acids in Chinese materia medica are formic acid, acetic acid, lactic acid, succinic acid, malic acid, tartaric acid and citric acid, which have an important effect on nutrition and physiology of human body.

Organic acid exists in the free state in plants or combines with Ca^{2+}, Na^+, K^+, Mg^{2+} and Ba^{2+}, etc., to form organic acid salts. Most organic acids have small molecular weight, easily dissolving in water. So, in order to avoid loss of organic acids, we should adopt the method of soaking little but moistening much when treating medicinal materials containing organic acids. However, if plants contain much soluble oxalate, they are often toxic. For example, Oxalis rubral (*Cujiang-cao*) can cause weakness, inhibition and even death. So in the course of processing, organic acid must be removed.

Heating can destroy certain organic acids. The organic acid with strong acidity has strong stimulation to oral cavities and stomachs. If drugs contain such organic acid, they should be heated to destruct the organic acid contents so as to meet the requirements of clinical medication. For example, stir – frying Fructus Crataegi (*Shanzha*) to brown can destroy some organic acids to decrease the acidity and the stimulation to gastrointestinal tracts. Qualitative change of organic acid will take place after being heated. For example, stir – frying coffee can destruct its chlorogenic acid to generate caffeic acid and quininic acid, and decrease the contents of tartaric acid, citric acid, malic acid and oxalic acid, to generate volatile acetic acid, propionic acid, butyric acid and valerian acid.

Some organic acids can react with alkaloid to form salts, which can increase the solubility of organic acids, and are beneficial to increase drugs' effects. So drugs containing alkaloids are often processed with Radix Glycyrrhizae (*Gancao*) to enhance its efficacy. The processing of Rhizoma Coptidis (*Huanglian*) and Fructus Evodiae (*Wuzhuyu*) are based on this principle too.

6. The Influence of Processing on Drugs Containing Grease

The main ingredient of grease is the long – chain fatty acid glyceride, mostly existing in plant seeds, with the function of moisturizing intestines, relaxing bowels, or causing diarrhea. Some has strong effect and certain toxicity.

Too much grease causes diarrhea, side – effects or toxicity, and they can be removed by heating or squeezing to guarantee the drugs' safety and effectiveness. For example, frosting Semen Platycladi (*Baiziren*) by defatting can reduce or eliminate its intestine – moistening effect. Frosting Semen Euphorbiae (*Qianjinzi*) by defatting can reduce its toxicity and moderate its properties. Frosting Semen Trichosanthis (*Gualouzi*) by defatting can remove the side – effects of inducing nausea and emesis so as to fit into patients with spleen and stomach deficiencies. The grease in Semen Ricini (*Bimazi*) can relieve swelling, eliminate toxicity, reduce diarrhea, and relieve stagnation of intestines. Stir – frying can denature the toxic protein of grease to avoid poisoning. Fructus Crotonis (*Badou*) oil is both an active and poisonous ingredient, when applying Fructus Crotonis (*Badou*) oil to clinical practice, we must control the dosage so as not to cause damage to patients.

7. The Influence of Processing on Drugs Containing Resin

Resin is a kind of complicated mixture, existing in the resin canal of plant tissues. When stimulated by injury or wound, plants can secrete resin to form solid or half – solids. Some are oleoresin, some are gum resin, and some are oleo – gum – resin. The resin has certain physiological effects and often used as antisepsis, expelling phlegm, antiinflammation, sedative, analgesic, antispasmodic, promoting blood circulation and hemostatic.

Generally, resin doesn't dissolve in water but dissolve in organic solvent like ethanol. Alcohol and vinegar are often used as supplement materials to process the drugs containing resin to increase its solubility and strengthen its effect. For example, processing Fructus Schisandrae (*Wuweizi*) with alcohol to improve its efficacy. Processing Resina Olibani (*Ruxiang*) and Myrrha (*Moyao*) with vinegar to strengthen their function of promoting blood and relieving pains.

Processing some resin drugs by heating can strengthen the efficacy, too. For example, processing gamboge (*Tenghuang*) at a high temperature can improve its antibacterial action. But the efficacy is weakened if the drug isn't heated properly. For example, stir – frying Resina Olibani (*Ruxiang*) and myrrh (*Moyao*) at too high temperature can weaken the efficacy due to the resin's denaturalization.

For the drugs in which the resin is not the active component or even has high toxicity, we may destruct part of the resin activity through heating so as to meet the clinical demands. For example, the resin of Semen Pharbitidis (*Qianniuzi*) has the purgative function which may be moderated by removing parts of resin through stir – frying.

8. The Influence of Processing on Drugs Containing Protein and Amino Acid

Protein is the most complicated substance in an organism. The hydrolysis of protein can create many kinds of amino acids, many of which are essential to the life activity of human beings. In addition, all the enzymes are protein. Protein is a kind of colloidal substance with a big molecular structure, most of protein can dissolve in water to form a colloidal solution and can't dissolve in water after being boiled for protein denaturation. Most of the pure amino acids are colorless crystals and can dissolve in water. To avoid the loss of active constituents, the drugs containing water – soluble amino acids shouldn't be soaked in water for long.

Heating can solidify and denature protein. Some amino acids aren't stable when being heated. So when using medicinal materials containing such substances, we should use them without any processing. For example, Radix Trichosanthis (*Tianhuafen*) and Apis Cerana Fabr (*Fengdu*), etc. Conversely, heating helps some drugs containing poisonous protein to be denatured to remove the toxicity. For example, Fructus Crotonis (*Badou*) and Semen Lablab Album (*Baibiandou*) should be heated to reduce their toxicity substantially. In accordance with these rules, when processing such drugs containing effective ingredients of glycoside as Radix Scutellariae (*Huangqin*) and Semen Armeniacae Amarum (*Kuxingren*), we should heat and boil them to destroy the activity of enzyme and protect the glycoside.

After being heated, proteins also can create some new substances to produce certain efficacy. For example, treating black soybean and yolk by dry distillation can create nitrogenous pyridines and porphyrins derivatives with detoxicating, antispasmodic, antipruritic, antibacterial and anti – allergy actions. With the existence of water, amino acid and monosaccharide react to form heterocycle compounds with special fragrance. For example, valine and sugar can react to form tasty light – brown melanoid; leucine and sugar can react to form heavy odor like bread. So stir – frying Fructus Hordei Germinatus (*Maiya*) can produce special fragrance which is beneficial to strengthen its actions of strengthening stomach and improving digestion.

Proteins can precipitate with many protein precipitant, such as tannin and heavy metal salts. So drugs containing protein shouldn't be processed together with drugs containing tannins. Acidity and basicity have great influences on stability and activity of proteins and amino acids, and it's important to process such drugs properly according to its property.

9. The Influence of Processing on Drugs Containing Sugar

Sugar is an important constituent in plants and accounts for 85% ~90% of organic substance in plants. It is the nourishing and sustaining substance of cells and tissues in plants. There are many types of sugars in plants including monosaccharide, polysaccharide and oligosaccharide. In the past, people didn't pay much attention to sugars. With the development of scientific research, people's attention to the biological activity of carbohydrate ingredient has been awakened. In the past few years, people discovered polysaccharides such as pachymaran and lentinan, etc. , which have apparent activities of improving the immune function of organism and a wide range of anti – cancer activity.

Monosaccharide and small molecule oligosaccharide easily dissolve in water, especially in hot water. Polysaccharide is hard to dissolve in water, but can be hydrolyzed into monosaccharide and oligosaccharide. So we'd better not use water to process drugs containing sugar. When having to soak them with water, we should adopt the little – soaking – but – much – moistening principle, particularly paying attention to the situation of heating together with water.

Sugar may combine with aglycone to form glycoside, namely the drugs containing glycoside can be hydrolyzed into sugars. For example, sweetness in Radix Rehmanniae Recens (*Dihuang*) and the content of reducing sugar in Radix Polygoni Multiflori (*Heshouwu*) increases after they are steamed, which is related to the change of carbohydrate.

10. The Influence of Processing on Drugs Containing Inorganic Compounds

Inorganic constituents widely exist in mineral drugs and shell drugs. There are also some inorganic salt existing in plants, such as sylvite, calcium, and magnesium, most of which combine with the organic acids in the tissue cells to form salt.

Mineral drugs are always processed by calcining or quenching with vinegar, which not only changes their physical properties and makes them easy to be crushed, thus being extracted easily, but also strengthens the efficacy due to their favorable gastrointestinal absorption, such as Magnetitum (*Cishi*) and Pyritum (*Zirantong*). Calcining the minerals containing crystallization water would make them lose the crystallization water, thus changing the efficacy of drugs, such as Gypsum Fibrosum (*Shigao*) and Alumen (*Mingfan*). In the process of heating and processing, certain constituents of the drugs maybe altered, accordingly generating new efficacy, such as Calamina (*Luganshi*). Calcining Calamina can change its main constituents, namely, turning zinc carbonate ($ZnCO_3$) into zinc oxide (ZnO), thereby having the effects of detoxifying, removing nebula to improve visual acuity, depriving dampness, alleviating itching and healing sores.

Treating the drugs containing such ingredients with water for a long time makes them lose water – soluble ingredients and inorganic salt, and decreases the efficacy of the drugs. For example, Spica Prunellae (*Xiakucao*) contains a great deal of sylvite. Its actions of promoting diuresis and lowering blood pressure decreases largely if soaking it in water for long.

Furthermore, people have made increasingly in – depth research in trace elements for they are essential to human health. The research shows there are 16 necessary trace elements and 25 trace elements closely linking to human bodies. For example zinc, it mainly exists in semen. People with zinc deficiency can't become taller and lose fecundity. Manganese deficiency causes mental retardation and sterility. Copper deficiency causes osteomalacia, dysplasia, joint deformity and albinism. Selenium can promote body immunity, and selenium deficiency causes a high incidence of cancer. Lithium can control the synthesis of catecholamine indirectly and adjust central nerve. These trace elements are thermally stable. Processing may destroy the organic components of drugs, thus making them be extracted easily, conducively bringing drugs' efficacy into full play.

In a word, various changes of physicochemical properties take place after drugs are processed with different methods. Until now, people understand some mechanism of processing, but most of the drugs' processing mechanism still need further studying. Guided by the theory of traditional Chinese medicine, and with the aid of modern scientific research methods, we analyze the mechanism of processing according to the influence of processing on the physicochemical properties of drugs so as to carry and develop the experiment knowledge of processing in the new historical circumstance.

第三章　中药炮制的目的及对药物的影响

第一节　中药炮制的目的

中药来源于植物、动物、矿物等，由于它们或质地坚硬、个体粗大，或含有泥沙杂质，或具有较大的毒副作用，一般不可直接用于临床，都要经过专门的加工炮制，使之成为饮片后才能应用。中药炮制的目的是多方面的，往往由于炮制方法不同，一种药物可同时具有多种作用，这些作用虽有主次之分，但彼此之间又有密切的联系。一般认为，中药炮制的目的有以下几个方面。

1. 降低或消除药物的毒性或副作用

有的药物虽有较好的疗效，但因毒性或副作用较大，临床应用不安全，通过炮制，可以降低其毒性或副作用。例如：草乌可通过浸渍，或漂洗，或清蒸，或单煮，或加入辅料共同蒸、煮降低其毒性或副作用。又如苍耳子、商陆等同样经过炮制后，可达到降低毒性的目的。

炮制也可除去或降低药物的副作用。汉代张仲景在《金匮玉函经》中明确指出：麻黄"生则令人烦，汗出不可止"，说明麻黄生用有"烦"和"出汗不止"的副作用，用时"皆先煮数沸"，便可除去其副作用。又如临床上遇到失眠、心神不安而又大便稀溏的病人，此时需用柏子仁宁心安神。但生柏子仁有滑肠通便的副作用，服后可使病人发生腹泻，此时可将柏子仁压去油脂制成柏子仁霜应用，以消除其副作用。

2. 改变或缓和药物的性能

中药是以寒、热、温、凉（即"四气"）和辛、甘、酸、苦、咸（即"五味"）来表示性能的。性味偏盛的药物，临床应用时往往会给病人带来一定的副作用。如太寒伤阳，太热伤阴，过辛耗气，过甘生湿，过酸损齿，过苦伤胃，过咸生痰。药物经过炮制，可以改变或缓和药物偏盛的性味，以达到改变药物作用的目的。唐代孙思邈在对孕妇使用桂枝时，为了防止"胎动"，特要求用"熬"法炮制后入药。明代罗周彦也曾提及枳壳"消食去积滞有麸炒，不尔气刚，恐伤元气"。又如麻黄生用辛散解表作用较强，经蜜炙炮制后，其所含具辛散解表作用的挥发油含量减少，辛散作用缓和。且炼蜜可润燥，能与麻黄起协同作用，故而止咳平喘作用增强。后人常用炒制、蜜炙等炮制方法来缓和药性，并总结出"甘能缓""炒以缓其性"的规律。

经炮制后，药物可改变其原有的药性，产生不同的临床疗效。如蒲黄，生品长于活血化瘀，炒制品可以止血；生甘草，性味甘凉，具有清热解毒的功效，但经蜜炙后，性味甘温，善于补脾益气、缓急止痛。因此，生品具有泻下作用的药物用作补益剂时，需蜜制。

3. 增强药物疗效

除配伍用药外，炮制也是增强药物疗效的有效方法。合理的炮制可增加药物的溶出速率并可以有效地促进药物的体内吸收而增强疗效。古人认为"决明子、莱菔子、白芥子、紫苏子、韭菜子、青葙子，凡药用子者俱要炒过，入药方得味出"。这是因为多数种子外有硬壳，其药效成分不易被煎出，经加热炒制后种皮爆裂，便于成分煎出。这就是后人"逢子必炒"的根据和用意。款冬花、紫菀等化痰止咳药经炼蜜炙制后，增强了润肺止咳的作用，这是因为炼蜜有甘缓益脾、润肺止咳之功，作为辅料被应用后与药物起协同作用，从而增强了疗效。现代实验证明，胆汁制南星能增强南星的镇痉作用，甘草制黄连可使黄连的抑菌效力提高数倍。可见药物经炮制可以从不同的方面增强其疗效。

4. 改变或增强药物的作用部位或趋向

中医对药物作用部位常以经络脏腑来表示，而对药物作用的趋向则是以升、降、沉、浮来表示。中药通过炮制，可以改变其作用趋向。同时，疾病的发病机制及症状也具有升降特性，如：咳嗽、哮喘、吐血等疾病呈现升的特性；而腹泻、出血、子宫遗尿症等病症则具有降的趋向。然而药物的作用趋势可以纠正生物体的这些机能紊乱。药物可通过炮制改变其归经，达到改变药物的作用位置或作用趋向的目的。如大黄苦寒，其性沉而不浮，经酒制后能引药上行。黄柏禀性至阴，气薄味厚，主降，但酒制后转降为升，清上焦之热。

临床上有时嫌一药入多经，会使其作用分散，通过炮制调整，可使其作用专一。例如柴胡入肝经、胆经、三焦，醋制之后入肝经作用增强。古人把它们总结为"生能升，熟能降""酒制升提""入盐走肾脏"。

5. 便于调剂和制剂

来源于植物类根、茎、藤、木、花、果、叶、草等的中药材，经水制软化，切制成一定规格的片、丝、段、块后，可便于调剂时分剂量、配药方。质地坚硬的矿物类、甲壳类及动物化石类药材，如自然铜、穿山甲、龟板、鳖甲、马钱子、阿胶，难于粉碎，通过煅、淬或砂烫、滑石粉烫等，在使药材从质坚变为酥脆的同时，也达到了增加其药效成分的溶出，有利于药物在体内的吸收等目的。

6. 便于储存保管

干燥药材减少它的含水量以防止霉变和虫蛀，使之更容易储存。煮，蒸，炒诸如昆虫和动物类药物可以杀死虫卵防止其孵化，如蒸桑螵蛸；蒸煮，炒制，灼烧种子类药材可以防止其萌发；有些含苷类成分的药物，如黄芩、苦杏仁等，经过加热处理，能促使其中与苷共存的酶失去活性，从而避免苷类成分在贮藏过程中被酶解而使疗效降低。

7. 矫臭矫味

中药中的某些动物类药材（如紫河车、海螵蛸）、树脂类药材（如乳香、没药）或其他有特殊不良气味的药物，往往为病人所厌恶，服后有恶心、呕吐、心烦等不良反应。为了便于服用，常用酒制、蜜制、水漂、麸炒、炒黄等方法炮制，能起到矫臭矫味的效果，如酒制乌梢蛇，麸炒僵蚕。

8. 洁净药物，确保质量

中药在采收、仓储、运输过程中常混有泥沙杂质或残留非药用部位和霉败品，因此必须经过严格的分离和洗刷，以保证临床用药的卫生和剂量的准确。例如根类药物的芦头（根上部之根茎部分）、皮类药材的粗皮（栓皮）、昆虫类药物的头足翅等常应除净。有的虽是一种植物，但由于部位不同，其药效作用亦不同。如麻黄，其茎能发汗，而其根却能止汗，故须分开。

第二节　炮制对药物化学成分的影响

药物的化学成分是药物发挥临床作用的物质基础。中药的化学成分组成相当复杂，对其中有效成分的状况尚有诸多不甚明了之处。可以认为中药的作用是综合性的，其所含各类成分之间有协同作用，也有对抗作用。中药炮制后，由于加热、水浸及酒、醋、药汁等辅料处理，无疑可使中药的化学成分发生一系列变化，一些成分含量增加了，另一些成分减少或消失了，或者产生新的化合物。因此，研究中药炮制前后化学成分的变化，对探讨中药炮制的作用和原理具有重要意义。由于许多中药的有效成分尚不明确，并且在此方面的研究没有充足的数据积累，因而，我们无法完整深入地讲述炮制对药物化学成分的影响。炮制对主要活性成分的影响大体有以下几方面：

1. 炮制对含生物碱类药物的影响

生物碱是一类含氮碱性有机化合物，味苦，具有生物活性。植物药和动物药都包含生物碱（如蟾酥）。

游离生物碱微溶于水，但易溶于乙醇、氯仿等有机溶剂或酸溶液中。大部分生物碱盐溶于水，但不溶或难溶于有机溶剂，因此酒和醋常被作为处理生物碱类药物的助溶剂。

酒既有极性溶剂的性质，又有非极性溶剂的性质，是一种良好的溶剂。中药化学成分的提取常使用乙醇，而酒就是具有稀醇性质的液体辅料。不论是游离生物碱或其盐类都能较易溶于酒。所以药物经过酒制后能提高生物碱的溶出率，从而提高药物的疗效。

醋是弱酸，能与游离生物碱结合成盐。生物碱的醋酸盐易被水溶出，增加水溶液中有效成分的含量，提高疗效。如延胡索主要有效成分是延胡索乙素、去氢延胡索甲素等，是具有止痛和镇静作用的生物碱，并以游离形式存在于药材中，难溶于水，但与醋酸结合生成醋酸盐后，在水中溶解度增加。所以延胡索经醋制后，其止痛效果增强。

生物碱在植物体中常与有机酸、无机酸生成复盐，如鞣酸盐、草酸盐等。它们是一种不溶于水的复盐，加入醋酸后，可以取代上述复盐中的酸类，形成可溶于水的醋酸盐复盐，增加了在水中的溶解度。

大多数生物碱不溶于水，但一些小分子生物碱如槟榔碱和一些季铵类如小檗碱溶于水。炮制过程中如有水洗、水浸等操作时，应尽量减少与水接触的时间，在切制时，也应采取"少泡多润"的原则，尽量减少在切片浸泡过程中生物碱的损失，以免影响疗效。

各种生物碱都有不同的耐热性。高温情况下某些生物碱不稳定，可产生水解、分解等变化。炮制常用煮、蒸、炒、烫、煅、炙等方法，改变生物碱的结构，以达到解毒、增效的目的。如乌头碱在高温条件下可水解成毒性小得多的乌头次碱或乌头原碱，因此炮制可以确保临床用药的安全性和有效性；而山豆根等药物所含生物碱遇热活性降低，而所含生物碱又是有效物质，因而炮制过程中应尽量减少热处理过程，以生用为宜。

2. 炮制对含苷类药物的影响

苷类成分在自然界中分布极广，广泛地存在于植物体中，尤其在果实、树皮和根部最多。

苷的溶解性能常无明显的规律，一般易溶于水或乙醇，有些苷也易溶于氯仿和乙酸乙酯，但难溶于乙醚和苯。溶解度还受糖分子数目和苷元所含极性基团的影响，若苷元极性基团多，则在水中的溶解度大，反之，在水中的溶解度就小。

酒作为炮制常用辅料，可提高含苷药物的溶解度，而增强疗效。由于苷类成分易溶于水，故中药在炮制过程中用水处理时应尽量"少泡多润"，以免苷类成分溶于水而流失，或发生水解而减少。常见者如大黄、甘草、秦皮等，均含可溶于水的各种苷，切制前用水处理时要特别注意。

含苷类成分的药物往往在不同细胞中含有相应的分解酶，在一定温度和湿度条件下可被相应的酶所分解，从而使有效成分减少，影响疗效。如槐花、苦杏仁、黄芩等含苷药物，采收后若长期放置，相应的酶便可分解芦丁、苦杏仁苷、黄芩苷，从而使这些药物疗效降低；花类药物所含的花色苷也可因酶的作用而变色脱瓣。所以含苷类药物常用炒、蒸、烘、焯或暴晒的方法破坏或抑制酶的活性，以保证药物有效物质免受酶解，保存药效。

苷类成分在酸性条件下容易水解，不但减低了苷的含量，也增加了成分的复杂性。因此，若苷类为药物的有效成分时，除医疗上有专门要求外，一般少用或不用醋处理。

3. 炮制对含挥发油类药物的影响

挥发油通常也是一种具有治疗作用的活性成分，挥发油也称精油，在常温下为易流动的油状液体，有香味和挥发性，一般指经水蒸气蒸馏所得到的挥发性油状成分的总称。挥发油一般具有芳香性，在常温下可以自行挥发而不留任何油迹，大多数比水轻，溶于多种有机溶剂及脂肪油中，在70%以上的乙醇中可全溶，在水中的溶解度极小。

很早以前，人们就知道在许多植物中含有挥发性的香气物质，并指出要尽量少加热或不加热。如《雷公炮炙论》中就对茵陈等注明"勿令犯火"。《本草纲目》在木香条下云："凡入理气药，不见火。若实大肠，宜面煨熟用。"所以凡含挥发性的药材应及时加工处理，干燥宜阴干，加水处理宜"抢水洗"，以免挥发油损失，对加热处理尤须注意。

但有些药物需要通过炮制以减少或除去挥发油，以达到医疗的需要。如麻黄，通过蜜炙加热处理，麻黄中具发汗作用的挥发油可减少1/2以上，而具有平喘作用的麻黄碱含量则基本未受影响，再加上蜂蜜的辅助作用，可使炙麻黄更适用于喘咳的治疗。又如苍术含挥发油较多，具有刺激性，即中医所指的"燥性"。据某些药物实验结果表明，炒炭可减少挥发油约80%，炒焦减少约40%，煨或土炒减少约20%，醋炙、酒炙、盐炙、米泔水制及麸炒减少约10%～15%，故应根据临床不同要求，选用不同的方法进行炮制。

药物经炮制后，不仅使挥发油的含量发生变化，有的也发生了质的变化。如颜色加深，折光率增大，或产生新的成分，有的还可改变药理作用。如荆芥炒炭后，从其所含挥发油中可检出9种生荆芥油所没有的成分，并且具有止血作用。肉豆蔻经煨制后，可增强其所含挥发油对家兔离体肠管收缩的抑制，从而产生实肠止泻作用。有些药物所含挥发油具有明显的毒性和强烈的刺激性，通过炮制后可大部分去除，有利临床应用。如乳香挥发油对胃有较强刺激性而致呕，生品多外用，经炮制去除大部分挥发油后，毒性和刺激性降低，可供内服。因而，某些药材中的挥发油具有明显的毒性和很强的刺激性，可以通过炮制满足临床应用要求。

挥发油在植物体内，多数是以游离状态存在，有的则以结合状态存在。对游离状态存在的薄荷、荆芥等宜在采收或喷润后迅速加工切制，不宜带水堆积久放，以免发酵变质，影响质量。有些药材所含挥发油是以结合状态存在于植物体内，则宜经堆积发酵后香气方可逸出，如厚朴必须经过埋藏发酵后，才能生产出优质的饮片来。

4. 炮制对含鞣质类药物的影响

鞣质是一类复杂的有酚类化合物，具有一定的活性，广泛地存在于植物中。鞣质具有止血、止泻、抑菌、保护黏膜等作用，常作为收敛剂，还作为生物碱及重金属中毒的解毒剂。

鞣质易溶于水，尤其易溶于热水中，因为其含有多元酚羟基，极性较强。所以在用水处理以鞣质为主要活性成分的药物时，要特别注意，比如地榆。

鞣质是一种强还原剂，在空气中易被氧气氧化而产生红色。槟榔、白芍等暴露在空气中颜色变红就是这个原因。鞣质在碱性溶剂中变色更快，在炮制过程中应特别注意。

鞣质一般对热稳定，在加热到很高的温度时其性质基本不变。例如，大黄含有致泻作用的蒽苷和收敛作用的鞣质，经酒蒸和炒炭后，蒽苷的含量明显减少，但鞣质的含量基本不变，因此致泻作用减弱而收敛作用相对增强。如果煎煮时间过长，蒽苷就会被破坏完全，大黄就不具有泻下作用反而会产生便秘。但是有一些鞣质的疗效会受炮制过程的高温影响，比如地榆炒炭的温度过高，其抑菌作用则大大减弱。因此，在炮制药物时要抓准炮制时间和火候。

鞣质遇到铁时会发生化学反应，生成墨绿色的鞣质铁盐沉淀。因此在切制含鞣质的药物时应用竹刀或钢刀，净洗时用木盘，煎煮时用砂锅以避免其与铁发生反应。

5. 炮制对含有机酸类药物的影响

有机酸广泛存在于植物细胞液中，尤其是在未成熟的肉质果实中。有机酸的含量会在果实成熟的过程中逐渐减少。中药材中常见的有机酸有甲酸、乙酸、乳酸、琥珀酸、苹果酸、酒石酸、枸橼酸，有机酸对人体营养和生理活动有重要的影响。

有机酸在植物体内一般呈游离状态存在，也可与钙、钠、钾、镁、钡等金属离子结合成有机酸盐。大多数有机酸的分子量小，易溶于水，因此在用水处理含有机酸类的药材时应采用少泡多润的方法，以避免有机酸的损失。但是如果植物含有较多的可溶性草酸盐时，往往有毒，比如酢浆草，动物食用酢浆草后会出现虚弱、抑制，甚至死亡。因此在炮制过程中必须将其除去。

加热可以破坏某些有机酸。具有强酸性的有机酸会对口腔和胃产生强烈的刺激性。因此，含有此类有机酸的药物在炮制时应加热破坏其有机酸的含量，以达到临床用药的要求。比如，山楂炒焦后，其内部有机酸被破坏，酸性降低而减少了对胃肠的刺激。有些有机酸的质量经加热后会发生转变。比如，咖啡经炒后其内绿原酸被破坏而生成咖啡酸和奎宁酸，同时减少酒石酸、枸橼酸、苹果酸、草酸，而生成挥发性的乙酸、丙酸、丁酸、缬草酸。

有些有机酸能与生物碱反应生成盐，这增加了有机酸的溶解度，有利于药物的疗效，因此常用甘草来炮制含有生物碱的药物以增强其药效。黄连、吴茱萸的炮制就是利用这个规律。

6. 炮制对含油脂类药物的影响

油脂的主要成分是长链脂肪酸的甘油酯，大多存在于植物的种子内，通常具有润肠通便或致泻的作用，有的作用竣烈，有一定的毒性。

油脂可以通过加热或压榨而除去以避免致泻或毒副作用，保证临床用药的安全有效。比如，柏子仁去油制霜能降低或消除滑肠作用；千金子去油制霜能减少毒性，缓和药性；瓜蒌仁去油制霜能消除恶心、呕吐等副作用，以适用于脾胃虚弱的患者；蓖麻子中的油脂具有减轻肿胀、消除毒性、减轻腹泻、减轻肠道阻滞等功能，炒制能使油脂中的毒性蛋白变性而失去活性，避免中毒；巴豆油既是有效成分又是有毒成分，用药时必须控制其用量以达到治疗而不伤人的目的。

7. 炮制对含树脂类药物的影响

树脂是一类成分复杂的混合物，存在于植物组织的树脂道中。植物体受到创伤刺激时就会分泌出树脂，并最终形成固体或半固体。有的为油树脂，有的为胶树脂，有的为油胶树脂。树脂具有一定的生理活性，经常被用于防腐、祛痰、消炎、镇静、镇痛、解痉、活血、止血。

通常树脂不溶于水而溶于有机溶剂，比如乙醇，酒和醋经常被作为辅料用于含树脂类药材的炮制，以增加其内树脂类成分的溶解度，增强药物的药效。如五味子的有效成分是树脂，用酒炮制五味子能提高其疗效；醋制乳香、没药能增强其活血止痛的作用。

通过加热炮制某些树脂类药物也可以增强其疗效。比如，藤黄经高温处理后其抑菌作用增强。但是，如果药物加热不当其疗效反而会降低。例如乳香、没药在炒制时若温度过高，则会使其变性，疗效降低。

对于树脂不是其有效成分或树脂毒性较大的药物，则可通过加热破坏部分树脂的活性，以满足临床需求。例如，牵牛子树脂具有泻下作用，经炒制后其部分树脂被破坏，泻下作用被减弱。

8. 炮制对含蛋白质，氨基酸类药物的影响

蛋白质是生物体内最复杂的物质。蛋白质水解能产生多种氨基酸，而其中很多种是人体生命活动必不可少的。另外，所有的酶都是蛋白质。蛋白质是一类大分子胶体物质，大多数可溶于水形成胶体溶液。煮沸后由于蛋白质变性而凝固，不再溶于水。纯净的氨基酸大多是无色的结晶体，能溶于水。含水溶性氨基酸的药材不应长时间浸泡在水中，以免有效成分流失而影响疗效。

加热可使蛋白质变性凝固。一些氨基酸在加热时不稳定，因此在使用含这类成分的药材时宜生药入药，比如天花粉、蜂毒等。一些含有毒性蛋白的药物可通过加热使蛋白质变性而达到去毒的目的，例如巴豆、白扁豆等，通过加热可以大幅度地降低其毒性。另外，根据这些规律，在炮制含苷类有效成分的药物时，如黄芪、苦杏仁，可以通过加热煮沸以达到杀酶保苷的目的。

蛋白质在加热后能产生新的物质从而产生一定的疗效。例如，经过干馏处理的黑大豆、鸡蛋黄能产生含氮的吡啶类、卟啉类衍生物而具有解毒、镇痉、止痒、抑菌、抗过敏作用。在有水存在的条件下，氨基酸能和单糖反应生成具有特异香味的环状化合物。例如，缬氨酸和糖能生成芳香可口的褐色类黑素，亮氨酸和糖能反应生成强烈的面包香味。所以，炒麦芽等能产生香味，增强其健脾消食的作用。

蛋白质能与许多蛋白质沉淀剂，比如鞣酸、重金属盐等反应产生沉淀，因此含蛋白质类的药物不能与含鞣质类的药物共同加工处理。酸度和碱度对蛋白质和氨基酸的稳定性和活性具有重大的影响，所以在加工炮制药物时应根据药物本身的性质加以恰当地处理。

9. 炮制对含糖类药物的影响

糖类成分在植物体内具有重要的意义，约占构成植物体有机物的 85%~90%。糖类是植物细胞与组织的重要营养物质和支持物质。糖类在植物体内的种类很多，包括单糖、多糖、寡糖。过去人们对药物中的糖类成分不甚关注，但随着科学研究的发展，人们对糖类成分的生理活性的注意力已被唤醒。在过去几年，人们发现多糖，如茯苓多糖、香菇多糖等具有明显的提高机体免疫功能和广泛的抗癌活性。

单糖和小分子寡糖易溶于水，尤其易溶于热水。多糖难溶于水，但能被水解成单糖和寡糖。因此在炮制含糖类成分的药物时最好不要用水，当某些药物必须用水时，应遵守少泡多润的原则，尤其要注意与水共同加热的情况。

糖可以和苷元结合形成苷，因此含糖苷类的药物能水解出糖。例如，地黄的甜度，何首乌还原糖的含量在经过蒸制后随之增加，这与糖类成分的变化有关。

10. 炮制对含无机化合物类药物的影响

无机成分大量存在于矿物类和贝壳类药物中。植物中也有无机盐类，如钾、钙、镁盐等，其中大多数是与组织细胞中的有机酸结合成盐。

矿物类药物通常采用煅烧或煅烧醋淬的方法，这不仅改变了其物理性状，使之易于粉碎，利于有效成分的溶出，而且有利于药物在胃肠道的吸收而增强疗效，例如磁石、自然

铜。含结晶水的矿物药经锻制后可使其内结晶水失去而改变药效，如石膏、明矾。在加热炮制过程中可以改变某些药物的成分从而产生新的治疗效果，例如炉甘石。煅烧炉甘石能改变其主要成分，使其从碳酸锌变成氧化锌，从而具有解毒、名目退翳、收湿止痒、敛疮的作用。

若长时间用水处理含此类成分的药物，会使药物的水溶性成分、无机盐损失而降低药物的疗效。例如，夏枯草含有大量的钾盐，如果长时间浸泡在水中则会使钾盐大量流失而使其利尿、降压功能大大减弱。

人们对微量元素的研究也日益深入，因为微量元素是人类健康不可或缺的重要物质。研究表明，有 16 种微量元素是人体必需的，25 种微量元素与人体有着密切的联系，比如锌。锌主要存在于精液中，缺乏锌人就会长不高并且失去生育能力；缺乏锰可引起智力低下和不育；缺乏铜会引起软骨病，发育不良，关节变形，白化病；硒可促进人体免疫，缺乏硒会引起癌症的发病率上升；锂可间接控制儿茶酚胺的合成，调节中枢神经。微量元素对热稳定，炮制工艺会破坏药物的有机成分，从而使微量元素更易溶出，有利于药物疗效的发挥。

总之，中药经过不同的加工炮制处理以后，其所含成分均有可能发生各种不同的变化，这些变化有些已被人们所了解，但绝大多数还有待深入研究。因此需要以中医药理论为指导，借助现代科学研究方法，依据炮制对药物理化性质的影响来分析炮制的机制，以在新的历史情境下传承和发展传统中药炮制的经验知识。

Chapter Four   The Classification and Adjuvant Materials of CMMP

Section One   Classifications of Processing

The classification of CMMP should reflect the intrinsic relationship among various professional skills of CMMP. Good classification does not only embody the inheritance of the traditional processing methods, but also benefit the modern research on CMMP. Therefore, such classification should have the property of systematization, integrality and scientificity, which can facilitate the study on CMMP, help teaching and guiding producing.

1. Master Lei's Seventeen Kinds of Processing Methods

In the *Ming* dynasty, Miu Xiyong summarized the processing methods in frontispiece of his book *Methods of Chinese Materia Medica Processing* (*Paozhidafa*), in which processing methods were classified into seventeen methods. They are roasting something with coat in fresh cinders, burning and baking, drying, roasting meat on the fire, roasting in fresh cinders, stir – frying, calcining, tempering and refining, processing, measuring size, refining powder with water, burning for a long time, planing with many blades, grinding and pounding, drying in the sun, and exposing to the air. Drugs should be processed by suitable methods to meet the clinical needs.

With the development of TCM, processing methods are no longer limited in the range of seventeen kinds of methods mentioned above. But this summary still has a certain influence on the practice of CMMP and it is also helpful for studying CMMP and consulting ancient documents.

2. Classification of Three Categories and Five Categories

Classification of three categories was put forward by Chen Jiamo in the *Ming* dynasty in his *Enlightenment on Materia Medica* (*Bencaomengquan*). It said that all the drugs were supposed to be processed with following methods: processing with fire (including methods of calcining, roasting drug with something covered on it, stir – frying with or without supplemental materials), processing with water (including methods of dipping, soaking and washing), processing with both water and fire (including methods of steaming and boiling). This classification can reflect the basic feature of processing.

But this classification could not involve all the processing methods. So classification of five categories was concluded later. The five categories include the methods of purifying, processing with water, processing with fire, processing with both water and fire, and other processing methods. It basically generalizes all the processing methods, which is more comprehensive compared to the three categories.

In modern times, processing methods are always classified into such three categories as cleaning, cutting and processing. This classification is adopted by *China Pharmacopoeia* (*Zhongguoyaodian*), as "general principles of drug processing" in appendix.

3. Classification Based on The Drug's Original Medicinal Part

In *Lei's Treatise on Preparation of Drugs*, various processing methods were listed dispersedly after the definition of drugs without any order. In *Formularies of the Bureau of People's Welfare Pharmacy* in the *Song* dynasty, processing methods were classified according to the nature and source of the drugs, such as metal, stone, grass, wood, water, fire, fruit, etc. But it is still limited in the category of Chinese materia medica.

Nowadays, national criterion and local criterion on processing often adopt the classification based on the drug's original medicinal part, in which drugs are classified into categories of roots and rhizomes, fruits and seeds, whole herbs, leaves, flowers, barks, vines, animals, minerals, etc. The processing methods are then narrated according to different categories of drugs. The advantage of this classification is the facilitation in consulting, but it cannot embody the systematization of processing technology.

4. Classification Combining Technology with Adjuvant Materials

Classification combining technology with adjuvant materials is developed from the classification of three categories and five categories. One is to give prominence to the action of adjuvant materials, taking adjuvant materials as the key link and technology as the supporting part, such as the method of processing with wine, honey, and ginger juice, etc. The methods of processing with wine are subdivided into stir – frying with wine, steaming with wine, and boiling with wine, etc. The other is to give prominence to the action of processing technology, taking technology as the key link and adjuvant materials as the supporting part, such as the methods of stir – frying, stir – frying with liquid adjuvant materials, calcining, steaming, boiling, and scalding, etc. The methods of stir – frying with liquid adjuvant materials are subdivided into the method of stir – frying with wine, vinegar, ginger juice, and honey, etc. This classification reflects the systematical and methodic features of CMMP. It involves both the advantage of technology and the advantage of classification based on adjuvant materials. It not only summarizes the whole procedure of processing technology but also expresses the action of adjuvant materials on drug. This kind of classification is generally adopted by the textbooks.

Section Two   Adjuvant Materials of Processing

The application of adjuvant materials of Chinese materia medica has a long history. It can go back to the period of Spring – autumn and Warring – states. The extensive use of adjuvant materials increases the flexibility of the drug's clinical application. Different adjuvant materials with different properties and functions exert different influence on processed drugs, which infers the close relation between drug's properties and adjuvant materials.

Adjuvant materials of preparation refer to all the additional materials except the main drug, which should have good chemical stability, would not react with the main drug and not affect the main drug's release, absorption and content determination in human body. But the concept of adjuvant materials of processing is different from the above meaning. Adjuvant materials of processing refer to the additional materials with supplementary action. They can improve the drug efficacy, reduce the drug's toxicity, or affect the drug's physicochemical property.

Now there are many kinds of adjuvant materials of processing, which can be classified into two categories: liquid adjuvant materials and solid adjuvant materials.

1. Liquid Adjuvant Materials

(1) Wine

The wine used for processing drugs often refers to the yellow wine and white spirits. The main components in wine are ethanol, esters, acids, etc.

Yellow wine is a Chinese beverage brewed from rice, wheat, or millet by using distiller's yeast. It contains 15% ~20% of ethanol with relative density of 0.98. It also contains sugar, ester, amino acid and mineral substance. It is generally the yellowish – brown and transparent liquid with special fragrance.

White spirits is another Chinese distilled beverage brewed from grains like rice, wheat, millet, potato, or Chinese sorghum with distiller's yeast. It contains 50% ~70% of ethanol with relative density of 0.82 ~0.92. It also contains acid, ester, aldehyde, etc. It is a kind of colorless transparent liquid with special fragrance and strong stimulation.

Wine is strongly hot in nature, sweet and pungent in flavor with the functions of promoting blood circulation for removing obstruction in collaterals, dispelling pathogenic wind and clearing away cold, guiding the drug's ascending tendency and modifying the terrible taste and fishy smell. Substances such as alkaloid, salts, glycosides, tannins, organic acid, volatile oil, resin, sugars and some pigments (chlorophyll or xanthophyll) can dissolve in wine easily. In addition, wine can increase the solubility of some inorganic components. For example, wine can react with some inorganic components ($MgCl_2$, $CaCl_2$, etc.) in plant to form crystal – like compounds called crystal alcohol ($MgCl_2 \cdot 6CH_3OH$, $CaCl_2 \cdot 4C_2H_5OH$), which dissolves in water easily, then, can increase the solubility.

Processing with wine can increase solubility of the drug's active ingredients and improve its therapeutic effectiveness. Processing the animal drug with wine can remove its terrible taste and fishy smell by volatilizing. The main components of the bad odor, such as trimethylamine and amino valeraldehyde, could dissolve in wine and volatile during processing. The aromatic substance of the esters in the wine can also modify its odor too. White spirits is often used for soaking drugs, while yellow wine is used for stir – frying drugs.

Wine should be transparent, without precipitates or impurities. It should have the special smell and taste of fragrance. It shouldn't ferment, spoilage or have abnormal taste. The content of alcohol in the wine should be consistent with the labeled concentration. The content of methyl alcohol should not be over 0.04g/100mL, the contents of sulfur dioxide should not be over 0.05g/kg, aflatoxin B_1 is not over 5μg/kg, bacteria is not over 50 per 1mL, the coliforms are not over 3 per 100mL.

Wine is often used as adjuvant materials for stir – frying, steaming and boiling. The drugs which are often processed with wine include Radix Scutellariae (*Huangqin*), Rhizoma Coptidis (*Huanglian*) Radix et Rhizoma Rhei (*Dahuang*), Radix Paeoniae Alba (*Baishao*), Radix Angelicae Sinensis (*Danggui*), etc.

(2) Vinegar

Vinegar includes rice vinegar, wheat vinegar, leaven vinegar and chemical vinegar. Now we often use edible vinegar (rice vinegar and other leaven vinegar) for processing. Chemical synthesis (vinegar concentrate) should not be used. The longer the storage time is, the better the vinegar is, and such vinegar is known as mature vinegar.

Vinegar is made from rice, wheat, grain sorghum and alcohol. Main component of vinegar is acetic acid with the content of 4% ~ 6%. It also contains vitamin, ash, succinic acid, oxalic acid, sorbose, etc.

Vinegar is sour, bitter in flavor and warm in nature with the functions of leading drug to the liver meridian, regulating vital energy, stopping bleeding, promoting diuresis, relieving edema, resolving toxins, removing blood stasis to stop pain and modifying the drug's terrible taste and fishy smell. Besides, vinegar can form salts with the free alkaloids in the drug, which increase the drug's solubility and improve its therapeutic effectiveness. Vinegar also has sterilizing and antiseptic function. It can kill pyogenic staphylococcus, salmonella, colibacillus and shigella dysenteriae within 30 minutes. In addition, vinegar can decrease the toxicity of Radix Phytolaccae (*Shanglu*), Herba Cirsii Japonici (*Daji*), Flos Genkwa (*Yuanhua*), etc. Vinegar can also form salt with trimethylamine to remove the drug's terrible odor.

Vinegar should be transparent, without turbid, suspended substance, precipitate and mold on the surface. It should have special smell of vinegar, not other bad or peculiar smell. Free acid shouldn't exist. Edible vinegar shouldn't be made by sulfuric acid, nitric acid, hydrochloric acid, etc. The total acid content shouldn't be less than 3.5%.

Vinegar is often used as adjuvant materials to process drugs like Rhizoma Corydalis (*Yanhusuo*), Radix Kansui (*Gansui*), and Radix Phytolaccae (*Shanglu*).

(3) Honey

The honey is brewed by the pollen collected by bees. There are many kinds of honey, among which jujube honey and litchi honey are considered to be better while buckwheat honey is bad for its dark color and terrible odor. The various kinds of honey differ greatly in chemical components due to different bees, nectar sources and environment. The main components of honey are fructopyranose and glucose with the content of 70%. Honey still contains a little saccharose, maltose, mineral, wax, oxygenates, enzyme, amino acid, vitamin, etc.

The differences in luster, color and fragrance of honey are determined by the nectar source, which can be identified by observing the shape of pollen grain under microscope.

The raw honey is cool in nature so it is often used to clear heat, but the cooked honey becomes warm in nature and is often used to strengthen the middle energizer. Honey is sweet in taste and mild in nature, which make it has the detoxifying function. It is often soft and moist to be used to moisturize dryness. It is absorbed slowly by body so it can alleviate pain. It also can be used to modify the bad odor. Neither cold nor dry, honey has mild nature, being suitable for varied diseases of twelve zang – fu organs. It thinks that honey has the function of harmonizing the property of different drugs.

But in processing, refined honey is more suitable. It is made by boiling the honey with proper amount of water, filtering it to remove the foam and impurities, and then concentrating.

Processing drugs with refined honey can improve the drug's efficacy, and also has the functions of detoxifying, harmonizing the actions of medicinal and modifying the drug's odor.

In spring and summer, honey is easy to ferment and foam to overflow or even break the container. So a few ginger pieces should be put in the container and cover it with a lid tightly to prevent fermentation. Honey should be stored in the dry and well ventilated place at 5℃ ~ 10℃. It is easy to absorb the smell of surroundings, so it shouldn't be stored near the source with fishy smell to avoid being polluted.

It is dangerous to store the honey in metal container, because the combination of ferrum and carbohydrate, zinc and organic acid can generate toxic substances. Zinc can dissolve in acid solvent, such as citric and acetic acid. If honey is stored in zinc container, zinc will combine with the organic acid in honey to form organic salt, which leads to zinc poisoning.

Honey should be a kind of semitransparent, glossy and dense liquid. It is fragrant and very sweet without bad smell. At 25℃, its relative density should be over 1.349. Starch and dextrin should not exist in it. The moisture content should not be over 25%, sucrose should not be over 8%, and reducing sugar should not be less than 64.0%.

Drugs like Radix Glycyrrhizae (*Gancao*), Herba Ephedrae (*Mahuang*), Radix Stemonae (*Baibu*), and Fructus Aristolochiae (*Madouling*) can be processed with honey.

(4) Salt Water

Salt water is a kind of transparent liquid by adding appropriate amount of water to dissolve salt crystals and then being filtered. Its main component is sodium chloride with a few of magnesium chloride, magnesium sulfate and calcium sulfate.

Salt is cold in nature and salty in flavor. It can strengthen tendons and bones, soften and resolve hard mass, clear away heat, cool the blood, resolve toxins, and modify the terrible odor. Processing the drug with salt water can change the drug's property and enhance its effects.

Salt should be white and salty, without visible impurities, bitterness, astringent and bad smell. The content of sodium chloride shouldn't be less than 96%. Both sulphate (counted with SO_4^{2-}) and magnesium shouldn't be more than 2%. The contents of barium, arsenic and lead shouldn't be more than 20mg/kg, 0.5mg/kg, 1mg/kg respectively.

Drugs like Cortex Eucommiae (*Duzhong*), Radix Morindae Officinalis (*Bajitian*), Fructus Foeniculi (*Xiaohuixiang*), Semen Citri Reticulatae (*Juhe*) and Semen Plantaginis (*Cheqianzi*) can be processed with salt water.

(5) Ginger Juice

Ginger juice is the juice made by pounding the rhizome of fresh ginger into pieces, or the yellowish white decoction of dried ginger after removing the residues. It has aroma. The main components of ginger juice are volatile oil, gingerol. It also contains various amino acid, starch, resin shaped substance, etc.

Ginger is pungent in flavor and warm in nature. It can relieve exterior syndrome by means of diaphoresis, warm the middle energizer, stop vomiting, dispel phlegm and resolve toxins. Processing the drug with ginger juice can restrain its coldness, improve its therapeutic effectiveness and reduce its toxicity.

Drugs like Caulis Bambusae in Taeniam (*Zhuru*), Rhizoma Pinelliae (*Banxia*), Rhizoma Coptidis (*Huanglian*), and Cortex Magnoliae Officinalis (*Houpo*) are often processed with ginger juice.

(6) Licorice Juice

Licorice juice, yellowish brown or dark brown, is the decoction of licorice after removing the residues. The main components of licorice are glycyrrhizin, liquiritin, reducing sugar, starch, glues, etc.

Licorice is sweet in flavor and neutral in nature. It can invigorate spleen and replenishing *qi*, clear away heat and relieve toxicity, dispel phlegm and relieve cough, relieve spasm and pain. Processing the drug with licorice juice can moderate its property and reduce its toxicity. The experiments show that licorice can be used, to a certain degree, to deal with the medicine or food poisoning, poisoning from internal metabolite and bacterial toxin. For example, it can counteract the toxicity of Cortex Meliae (*Kulianpi*) and Radix Sophorae Tonkinensis (*Shandougen*). It can also reduce the side - effects of streptomycin and furadantin. The detoxifying mechanism of licorice is as following. Firstly, the glycyrrhizin is able to absorb the toxic substances. Secondly, glycyrrhizin can be hydrolyzed to form glucuronic acid, which can be combined with the toxic compounds with hydroxyl and carboxyl. The product of this process is uneasy to be absorbed in vivo and then ejected with urine. Finally, glycyrrhizin can also strengthen the liver's function of detoxification. In addition, liquiritin, the extract of licorice, is a kind of surface active agent. After being shaken, it will produce stable foam to reduce the surface tension and increase the solubility of some materials which are difficult to dissolve in water. In the prescription of TCM, licorice is often used as the guiding drug to harmonize the actions of other medicinal in a formula. And it also can be used to increase the solubility during processing and decoction.

Drugs like Radix Polygalae (*Yuanzhi*), Rhizoma Pinelliae (*Banxia*) and Fructus Evodiae (*Wuzhuyu*) are often processed with licorice juice.

(7) Black Soybean Juice

Black soybean juice, black and turbid, is the decoction of the black seeds of soybeans. The residues in the decoction should be removed. Black soybean contains protein, fat, vitamin, pigment, starch, etc.

Black soybean is sweet in flavor and mild in nature. It can active blood circulation and induce diuresis, dispel wind, remove the toxic substances, and nourish liver and kidney. Processing the drug with black soybean juice can improve its therapeutic effectiveness and reduce its toxicity or side effects.

Drugs like Radix Polygoni Multiflori (*Heshouwu*) is often processed with black soybean juice.

(8) Rice – washed Water

Rice – washed water is the water in which rice has been washed for the second time. It contains a little starch and vitamin. And it should be prepared just before using because it is easy to ferment.

Rice – washed water is sweet in flavor and cool in nature, non – toxic. It can invigorate vital energy, relieve vexation and thirst, and resolve toxins. Because this kind of water can absorb oil, it is often used to soak the greasy drug to remove part of grease from the drug. In doing so, it can decrease the drug's pungent flavor and drastic properties and strengthen the functions of replenishing the spleen and strengthening the middle energizer. Drugs like Rhizoma Atractylodis (*Cangzhu*) and Rhizoma Atractylodis Macrocephalae (*Baizhu*) are often processed with it.

Nowadays, for mass production, it is difficult to collect rice – washed water. Therefore, it is often replaced by the mixture of 2kg rice flour and 100kg water.

(9) Bile

Bile refers to the fresh bile of cattle, pig and sheep. It is greenish brown, slightly transparent, and sticky, with special fishy smell. Its main components are sodium cholate, bile pigment, mucin, lipid, inorganic salts, etc.

Bile is bitter in flavor and strongly cold in nature. It can clear liver fire for improving eyesight, promote gallbladder function and bowel movements, resolve toxins and alleviate edema and moisten dryness. Processing the drug with bile can reduce the drug's toxicity and drastic property to improve its therapeutic effectiveness. It is mainly used to process Rhizoma Arisaematis (*Tiannanxing*).

(10) Sesame Oil

Sesame oil is an edible oil extracted from the dry matured seeds of sesame, cold pressed or hot pressed. Its main components are linoleic acid glyceride, sesamin, etc.

Sesame oil is sweet in flavor and slightly cold in nature. It can clear away heat, moisten dryness and promote tissue regeneration. Because of its high boiling point, sesame oil is often used to process hard or poisonous drugs to make them crisp and decrease their toxicity. The sesame oil mixed with impurities or the spoilage shouldn't be used. Drugs like Semen Strychni (*Maqianzi*), Pheretima (*Dilong*) and Os Pardi (*Baogu*) are often processed with sesame oil.

Other liquid adjuvant materials include the decoction of Fructus Evodiae (*Wuzhuyu*), radish juice, suet oil, turtle blood, limewater, etc.

2. Solid Adjuvant Materials

(1) Rice

Rice is the kernel of paddy, Gramineae plants. Its main components are starch, protein, fat and mineral substance. It also contains vitamin B, various organic acid and sugar.

Rice is sweet in flavor and neutral in nature. It can strengthen the middle energizer and benefit vital energy, invigorate spleen and regulate the stomach, relieve vexation and quench thirst, relieve diarrhea and dysentery. Processing the drug with rice can enhance the drug's effect while decrease its stimulation and toxicity. Therefore, rice or glutinous rice is often used to process drugs like Mylabris (*Banmao*), Radix Codonopsis (*Dangshen*), etc.

(2) Wheat Bran

Wheat bran is the brownish yellow episperm of wheat. It mainly contains starch, protein and vitamin.

It is sweet and tasteless in flavor and plain in nature. It can regulate the middle energizer and benefit the spleen. Processing the drug with wheat bran can moderate drugs' drastic property, improve its therapeutic effectiveness, remove its bad smell, and make the color and luster well distributed. Besides, wheat bran also can be used to absorb oil and it could be used as supplementary material for ash – roasting. Drugs like Rhizoma Atractylodis (*Cangzhu*) and Rhizoma Atractylodis Macrocephalae (*Baizhu*) are often processed with wheat bran.

(3) Alum

Alum is the irregularly lump – shaped crystal which is refined from alumen of trigonal system. This crystal is colorless, transparent or semitransparent, with glass – like luster and crisp in texture. It is slightly sour and astringent in flavor and can dissolve in water easily. Its main component is water – containing aluminium potassium sulfate.

Alum is sour in flavor and cold in nature. It can resolve toxins, dispel phlegm and kill parasite, astringe and deprive dampness, it also has antiseptic function. Processing the drug with alum can prevent the drug from rotting, decrease its toxicity and improve its therapeutic effectiveness. Drugs like Rhizoma Pinelliae (*Banxia*) and Rhizoma Arisaematis (*Tiannanxing*) are often processed with alum.

(4) Bean Curd

Bean curd is the soft white blocks made by grinding the seeds of soybeans and processing with special technic. It mainly contains protein, vitamin and starch.

Bean curd is sweet in taste and cool in nature. It can strengthen vital energy and regulate the middle energizer, promote the production of body fluid and moisturize dryness, clear heat and relieve toxins. Bean curd has strong actions of precipitation and absorption. Processing the drug with bean curd can reduce its toxicity and clear away the dirt. Drugs like Garcinia morella Desv (*Tenghuang*), Margarita (*Zhenzhu*) and Sulfur (*Liuhuang*) are often processed with bean curd.

(5) Soil

Soil refers to the soil in kitchen range, loess and red halloysite. The soil in kitchen range looks like scorched earth, which is blackish brown with sootiness fragrance. Its main components are silicate, calcium salts and many alkaline oxides.

The soil in kitchen range is pungent in taste and warm in nature. It can warm the middle energizer and harmonize stomach, stop bleeding and vomiting, astringe the intestines and check diarrhea. Processing the drug with soil can decrease drugs' stimulation and improve its therapeutic effectiveness. Drugs like Rhizoma Atractylodis Macrocephalae (*Baizhu*), Radix Angelicae Sinensis (*Danggui*), and Rhizoma Dioscoreae (*Shanyao*) are often processed with soil.

(6) Clam Powder

Clam powder is the grayish white powder made by calcining and smashing the shell of Meretrix meretrix Linnaeus (*Wenge*) and Cyclina sinensis Gmelin (*Qingge*) etc. Its main components are calcium oxide.

Clam powder is salty in flavor and cold in nature. It can clear heat, promote dampness, dispel phlegm and soften hardness. Processing the drug with clam powder can remove drug's fishy smell and improve its therapeutic effectiveness. It is mainly used for stir – frying Colla Corii Asini (*E'jiao*).

(7) Talcum Powder

Talcum powder is the fine powder made by cleaning, grinding and drying the talcum of silicate ore of monoclinic system, mainly containing hydrated magnesium silicate. This kind of fine powder has a soapy feel and appears to be white or nearly white in color.

It is sweet in taste and cold in nature. It can promote diuresis and clear summer heat. It is often used as heat transfer to make the drug heated evenly. Drugs like Corium Erinacei (*Ciweipi*) are often stir – fried with talcum powder.

(8) River Sand

Before use, river sand should be sieved and selected with average size, washed and removed from the impurities, and then dried in the sun for use. River sands are usually stir – fried with hard drug as the heat transfer because they are easy to reach high temperature and have good diathermancy. Processed with river sand, the drug can be heated evenly and become crisp, which make it easy for crushing and decoction. In addition, the processing can also remove the toxicity and non – medicinal parts of the drug. Drugs like Semen Strychni (*Maqianzi*), Squama Manitis (*Chuanshanjia*), Carapax Trionycis (*Biejia*) and Carapax et Plastrum Testudinis (*Guijia*) are often stir – fried with sand.

(9) Cinnabar

Cinnalar is the mineral Cinnabaris of trigonal system, which contains mercuric sulfide.

Cinnabar is sweet in taste and slightly cold in nature. It can relieve convulsions, tranquilization, and resolve toxins. Drugs such as Indian bread (*Fuling*), Poria cum Radix Pini (*Fushen*) and Radix Polygalae (*Yuanzhi*) are often processed by stirring with cinnabar.

第四章 中药炮制的分类及辅料

第一节 炮制的分类方法

中药炮制的分类，应反映中药炮制专业技术内在的有机联系，既要体现对传统炮制方法的继承，又要有利于炮制的现代研究。因此，要求分类必须具有系统性、完整性和科学性，便于学习、掌握中药炮制的内容，有助于教学和指导生产。

1. 雷公炮炙十七法

明代缪希雍在《炮炙大法》卷首把当时的炮制方法进行了归纳，云："按雷公炮炙法有十七：曰炮、曰燀、曰煿、曰炙、曰煨、曰炒、曰煅、曰炼、曰制、曰度、曰飞、曰伏、曰镑、曰搬、曰曬、曰曝、曰露是也，用者宜如法，各尽其宜。"

随着中医药的发展，炮制方法不断增多并日趋完善，已远远超出了十七法的范围，但其对中药炮制的基本操作至今仍有一定的影响。尤其对学习中药炮制和查阅古代文献有一定的帮助。

2. 三类和五类分类法

三类分类法是明代陈嘉谟在《本草蒙筌》中提出的："凡药制造……火制四：有煅、有炮、有炙、有炒之不同；水制三：或渍、或泡、或洗之弗等；水火共制造者：若蒸、若煮而有二焉，余外制虽多端，总不离此二者。"此种分类方法基本能反映出炮制的特色。

由于火制、水制、水火共制尚不能包括中药炮制的全部内容，后来总结归纳了五类分类法。五类分类法包括：修治、水制、火制、水火共制、其他制法，这样就基本概括了所有的炮制方法，相比三类分类法更全面。

近代，依据中药炮制的工艺分为净制、切制和炮炙三大类，《中国药典》一部附录收载的"药材炮制通则"就是采用这种分类方法。

3. 药用部位分类法

中药炮制专著《雷公炮炙论》，全书将炮制方法散列于各药之后，无规律可循。至宋代《太平惠民和剂局方》，把炮制依据药物来源属性的金、石、草、木、水、火、果等分类，但仍局限于本草学的范畴。

现今，全国中药炮制规范及各省市制订的炮制规范，大多以药用部位的来源进行分类，即：根及根茎类，果实、种子类，全草类，叶类，花类，皮类，藤木类，动物类，矿物类等，在各种药物项下再分述各种炮制方法。此种分类方法的优点便于具体药物的查阅，但体现不出炮制工艺的系统性。

4. 工艺与辅料相结合的分类法

工艺与辅料相结合的分类方法是在三类、五类分类法的基础上发展起来的。其一法是突出辅料对药物所起的作用，以辅料为纲，以工艺为目的的分类法，如分为酒制法、蜜制法、姜制法等。在酒制法中再分为酒炙、酒蒸、酒煮等。其二法是突出炮制工艺的作用，以工艺为纲，以辅料为目的的分类法，如分为炒、炙、煅、蒸、煮、燀等。在炙法中再分为酒炙法、醋炙法、姜炙法、蜜炙法等。这种分类方法能较好地体现中药炮制工艺的系统性、条理性，它吸收了工艺法的长处，采纳了辅料分类的优点，既能体现整个炮制工艺程序，又便于叙述辅料对药物所起的作用，一般多为教材所采用。

第二节   中药炮制辅料

中药炮制应用辅料的历史非常久远，大约在春秋战国时期即开始应用。辅料的广泛应用增加了临床用药的灵活性。由于辅料品种不同，更由于各种辅料性能和作用不同，在炮制药材时所起的作用也各不相同，提示了药性与辅料之间的密切联系。

制剂辅料是除主药以外的一切附加物料的总称，它必须具有较高的化学稳定性，不与主药起反应，不影响主药的释放、吸收和含量测定。但炮制辅料的概念则不相同，是指具有辅助作用的附加物料，它对主药可起到增强疗效，或降低毒性，或影响主药的理化性质等作用。

目前常用的中药炮制辅料种类较多，一般可分为液体辅料和固体辅料两大类。

1. 液体辅料

（1）酒

用以制药的酒有黄酒、白酒两大类，主要成分为乙醇、酯类、酸类等物质。

黄酒为米、麦、黍等用曲酿制而成，含乙醇15%～20%，相对密度约0.98，尚含糖类、酯类、氨基酸、矿物质等。一般为棕黄色透明液体，气味醇香特异。

白酒为米、麦、黍、薯类、高粱等用曲酿制并经蒸馏而成，含乙醇50%～70%，相对密度0.82～0.92，尚含酸类、酯类、醛类等成分。一般为无色澄明液体，气味醇香特异，且有较强的刺激性。

酒性大热，味甘、辛。能活血通络，祛风散寒，行药势，矫味矫臭。生物碱及盐类、苷类、鞣质、有机酸、挥发油、树脂、糖类及部分色素（叶绿素、叶黄素）等皆易溶于酒。此外，酒还能提高某些无机成分的溶解度，如酒可以和植物体内的一些无机成分（$MgCl_2$、$CaCl_2$等）形成结晶状的分子化合物，称结晶醇（$MgCl_2 \cdot 6CH_3OH$、$CaCl_2 \cdot 4C_2H_5OH$），结晶醇易溶于水，故可提高其溶解度。

药物经酒制后，有助于有效成分的溶出而增加疗效。动物的腥膻气味为三甲胺、氨基戊醛类等成分，酒制时此类成分可随酒挥发而除去。酒中含有酯类等醇香物质，可以矫味矫臭。浸药多用白酒，炙药用黄酒。

酒应透明，无沉淀或杂质，具有酒特有的芳香气味，不应有发酵、酸败或异味。含醇量应符合标示浓度，甲醇量不得超过 0.04g/100mL，二氧化硫或残留量不超过 0.05g/kg，黄曲霉素 B_1 不超过 5μg/kg，细菌数不超过 50 个/mL，大肠菌群不超过 3 个/100mL。

酒多用作炙、蒸、煮等辅料，常用酒制的药物有黄芩、黄连、大黄、白芍、当归等。

（2）醋

醋有米醋、麦醋、曲醋、化学醋等多种。如今，炮制用醋多为食用醋（米醋或其他发酵醋），化学合成品（醋精）不应使用。醋存放时间越长越好，称为"陈醋"。

醋是以米、麦、高粱以及酒精等酿制而成。主要成分为醋酸，占 4% ~6%，尚有维生素、灰分、琥珀酸、草酸、山梨糖等。

醋味酸、苦，性温。具有引药入肝、理气、止血、行水、消肿、解毒、散瘀止痛、矫味矫臭等作用。同时，醋具酸性，能与药物中所含的游离生物碱等成分结合成盐，从而增加其溶解度而易煎出有效成分，提高疗效。醋具有杀菌防腐作用，它能在 30 分钟内杀死化脓性葡萄球菌、沙门菌、大肠杆菌、痢疾杆菌等。醋能使商陆、大戟、芫花等药物毒性降低而有解毒作用。醋能和具腥膻气味的三甲胺类成分结合成盐而无臭气，故可除去药物的腥臭气味。

醋应澄明，不浑浊，无悬浮物及沉淀物，无霉花浮膜，具醋特异气味，无其他不良气味与异味。不得检出游离酸，防止用硫酸、硝酸、盐酸等矿酸来制造食醋。总酸量不得低于 3.5%。

常用醋制的药物有延胡索、甘遂、商陆等。

（3）蜂蜜

为蜜蜂采集花粉酿制而成，品种比较复杂，以枣花蜜、荔枝蜜等质量为佳，荞麦蜜色深有异臭，质差。蜂蜜因蜂种、蜜源、环境等不同，其化学组成差异较大。主要成分为果糖、葡萄糖，两者约占蜂蜜的 70%，尚含少量蔗糖、麦芽糖、矿物质、蜡质、含氧化合物、酶类、氨基酸、维生素等物质。

蜂蜜的色泽、香气差异取决于生蜜的花粉来源，可借助显微镜观察花粉粒的形状进行鉴定。

蜂蜜生则性凉，故能清热；熟则性温，故能补中；以其甘而平和，故能解毒；柔而濡泽，故能润燥；缓可去急，故能止痛；气味香甜，故能矫味矫臭；不冷不燥，得中和之气，故十二脏腑之病，无不宜之。因而认为蜂蜜有调和药性的作用。

中药炮制常用的是炼蜜，即将生蜜加适量水煮沸，滤过，去沫及杂质，稍浓缩而成。

用炼蜜炮制药物，能与药物起协同作用，增强药物疗效或起解毒、缓和药物性能、矫味矫臭等作用。

蜂蜜春夏易发酵、易起泡沫而溢出或挤破容器，可加少许生姜片，盖严，能起一定的预防作用。应贮存在 5℃ ~10℃干燥通风处，防止发酵。蜂蜜易吸附外界气味，不宜存放在有腥臭气源附近，以免污染。

用金属容器贮藏蜂蜜是有危险的，因为铁与蜂蜜中的糖类化合物作用，锌与蜂蜜中的有机酸作用，均可生成有毒物质。锌能溶于酸性溶液中，如柠檬酸、醋酸等，若在锌容器内贮藏蜂蜜，锌与蜂蜜中的有机酸生成有毒的有机酸盐，食后便发生锌中毒。

蜂蜜应是半透明、带光泽、浓稠的液体，气芳香，味极甜，不得有不良的异味。室温（25℃）相对密度应在 1.349 以上。不得有淀粉和糊精，水分不得超过 25%，蔗糖不得超过 8%，还原糖不得少于 64%。

常用蜂蜜炮制的药物有甘草、麻黄、百部、马兜铃等。

（4）食盐水

为食盐的结晶体，加适量水溶化，经过滤而得的澄明液体。主含氯化钠，尚含少量的氯化镁、硫酸镁、硫酸钙等。

食盐性味咸寒，能强筋骨、软坚散结、清热、凉血、解毒，并能矫味。药物经食盐水制后，能改变药物的性能，增强药物的作用。

食盐应为白色，味咸，无可见的外来杂物，无苦味、涩味，无异臭。氯化钠含量 ≥ 96%，硫酸盐（以 SO_4^{2-} 计）≤ 2%，镁 ≤ 2%，钡 ≤ 20mg/kg，砷 ≤ 0.5mg/kg，铅 ≤ 1mg/kg。

常以食盐水炮制的药物有杜仲、巴戟天、小茴香、橘核、车前子等。

（5）生姜汁

为姜科植物鲜姜的根茎经捣碎取的汁；或用干姜加适量水共煎去渣而得的黄白色液体。姜汁有香气，其主要成分为挥发油、姜辣素，另外尚含有多种氨基酸、淀粉及树脂状物。

生姜味辛，性温。升腾发散而走表，温中，止呕，开痰，解毒。药物经姜汁制后能抑制其寒性，增强疗效，降低毒性。

常以姜汁制的药物有竹茹、半夏、黄连、厚朴等。

（6）甘草汁

为甘草饮片水煎去渣而得的黄棕色至深棕色的液体。甘草主要成分为甘草甜素及甘草苷、还原糖、淀粉及胶类物质等。

甘草味甘，性平。具补脾益气、清热解毒、祛痰止咳、缓急止痛的作用。药物经甘草汁制后能缓和药性，降低毒性。实验证明，甘草对药物中毒、食物中毒、体内代谢物中毒及细菌毒素都有一定的解毒作用。如能解苦楝皮、山豆根的毒，还能降低链霉素、呋喃坦啶的毒副作用。其解毒机理一般认为：甘草甜素对毒性物质有某种吸附作用；甘草甜素水解后生成葡萄糖醛酸，可与有羟基或羧基的毒物生成在体内不易被吸收的产物，分解物从尿中排出；此外，甘草甜素还能增强肝脏的解毒功能。甘草苷系表面活性剂，甘草浸出液，振摇之后产生稳定的泡沫，减低表面张力，能增加其他不溶于水物质的溶解度。中医处方中常用甘草为药引，调和诸药，在炮制和煎煮过程中亦起到增溶的作用。

常以甘草汁制的药物有远志、半夏、吴茱萸等。

（7）黑豆汁

为大豆的黑色种子加适量水煮熬去渣而得的黑色混浊液体。黑豆含蛋白质、脂肪、维生素、色素、淀粉等物质。

黑豆味甘，性平。能活血、利水、祛风、解毒、滋补肝肾。药物经黑豆汁制后能增强药物的疗效，降低药物毒性或副作用等。

常以黑豆汁制的药物有何首乌等。

（8）米泔水

为第二次的淘米水，其中含少量淀粉和维生素等。因易酸败发酵，应临用时收集。

米泔水味甘，性凉，无毒。能益气，除烦，止渴，解毒。米泔水对油脂有吸附作用，常用来浸泡含油质较多的药物，以除去部分油质，降低药物辛燥之性，增强补脾和中的作用。常以米泔水制的药物有苍术、白术等。

目前因米泔水不易收集，大生产也有用 2kg 米粉加水 100kg，充分搅拌代替米泔水用者。

（9）胆汁

系牛、猪、羊的新鲜胆汁，为绿褐色、微透明的液体，略有黏性，有特异腥臭气，主要成分为胆酸钠、胆色素、黏蛋白、脂类及无机盐类等。

胆汁味苦，性大寒。能清肝明目，利胆通肠，解毒消肿，润燥。与药物共制后，能降低药物的毒性或燥性，增强疗效。主要用于制备胆南星。

（10）麻油

为胡麻科植物脂麻的干燥成熟种子经冷压或热压所得的油脂，主要成分为亚油酸甘油酯、芝麻素等。

麻油味甘，性微寒。能清热，润燥，生肌。因沸点较高，常用以炮制质地坚硬或有毒药物，使之酥脆，降低毒性。凡混入杂质或酸败者不可用。常用麻油制的药物有马钱子、地龙、豹骨等。

其他的液体辅料还有吴茱萸汁、萝卜汁、羊脂油、鳖血、石灰水等。

2. 固体辅料

（1）稻米

稻米为禾本科植物稻的种仁。主要成分为淀粉、蛋白质、脂肪、矿物质等，尚含少量的 B 族维生素、多种有机酸及糖类。

稻米味甘，性平。能补中益气，健脾和胃，除烦止渴，止泻痢。与药物共制，可增强药物功能，降低刺激性和毒性。中药炮制多选用大米或糯米。常用米制的药物有斑蝥、党参等。

（2）麦麸

麦麸为小麦的种皮，呈褐黄色。主含淀粉、蛋白质及维生素等。

麦麸味甘、淡，性平，能和中益脾。与药物共制能缓和药物的燥性，增强疗效，除去药物不良气味，使药物色泽均匀一致。麦麸还能吸附油质，亦可作为煨制的辅料。常以麦麸制的药物有苍术、白术等。

（3）白矾

又称明矾，为三方晶系明矾矿石经提炼而成的不规则的块状结晶体，无色，透明或半透明，有玻璃样色泽，质硬脆易碎，味微酸而涩，易溶于水，主要成分为含水硫酸铝钾。

白矾味酸，性寒。能解毒，祛痰杀虫，收敛燥湿，防腐。与药物共制后，可防止腐烂，降低毒性，增强疗效。常以白矾制的药物有半夏、天南星等。

（4）豆腐

豆腐为大豆种子粉碎后经特殊加工制成的乳白色固体，主含蛋白质、维生素、淀粉等物质。

豆腐味甘，性凉。能益气和中，生津润燥，清热解毒。豆腐具有较强的沉淀与吸附作用，与药物共制后可降低药物毒性，去除污物。常与豆腐共制的药物有藤黄、珍珠、硫黄等。

（5）土

中药炮制常用的是灶心土（伏龙肝），也可用黄土、赤石脂等。灶心土呈焦土状，黑褐色，有烟熏气味。主含硅酸盐、钙盐及多种碱性氧化物。

灶心土味辛，性温。能温中和胃，止血，止呕，涩肠止泻等。与药物共制后可降低药物的刺激性，增强药物疗效。常以土制的药物有白术、当归、山药等。

（6）蛤粉

为帘蛤科动物文蛤、青蛤等的贝壳，经煅制粉碎后的灰白色粉末。主要成分为氧化钙等。

蛤粉味咸，性寒。能清热利湿，化痰，软坚。与药物共制可除去药物的腥味，增强疗效。主要用于烫制阿胶。

（7）滑石粉

为单斜晶系硅酸盐类矿物滑石经精选净化、粉碎、干燥而制得的细粉。主要含有水合硅酸镁。本品为白色或类白色、微细的粉末，手摸有滑腻感。

滑石粉味甘，性寒。能利尿，清热，解暑。中药炮制常用滑石粉作中间传热体拌炒药物，可使药物受热均匀。常用滑石粉烫炒的药物有刺猬皮等。

（8）河砂

筛取粒度均匀适中的河砂，淘净泥土，除尽杂质，晒干备用。中药炮制常用河砂作中间传热体拌炒药物，主要取其温度高、传热快的特点，可使坚硬的药物受热均匀，经砂炒后药物质地变松脆，以便粉碎和利于煎出有效成分。另外砂烫炒还可以破坏药物毒性成分，易于除去非药用部位。常以砂烫炒的药物有马钱子、穿山甲、鳖甲、龟甲等。

（9）朱砂

为三方晶系硫化物类矿物辰砂，主要成分为硫化汞。

朱砂味甘，性微寒。具有镇惊、安神、解毒等功效。常用朱砂拌制的药材有茯苓、茯神、远志等。

Chapter Five Quality Control and Storage

Section One Quality Control

1. Purity

（1）Definition

Purity here refers to the limit for the impurities and non – medicinal parts in processed products.

（2）Requirements

According to *General Quality Standards for Traditional Chinese Medicine Decoction Pieces* (hereinafter referred to as *General Quality Standards*), issued by State Administration of Traditional Chinese Medicine, the processed products should not have substances like sediment, ash, mildew products, pieces bitten by insect, foreign substances and non-medicinal parts. In the processed products from fruit, seed, herbs and resin, the content of medicine dusts and non – medicinal parts should be less than 3%; in those from root, tuber, leaf, flower, rattan, skin, animal, mineral, bacteria and alga, less than 2%; in products that are stir – fried without adjuvant materials or fried with rice, products fried with wine, vinegar or salt water, fermented products and germinated products, the content should be less than 1%.

2. Shape and Size

（1）Shape of Pieces

According to *Chinese Pharmacopoeia* and *National Traditional Chinese Medicine Preparation Standards*, sliced pieces should have uniform thickness, bright color and smooth surface, without contamination or extensive diffusion of oil. According to *General Quality Standards*, the amount of special – shaped pieces should be less than 10%; the thickness deviation between the extremely thin slices and standard pieces should be less than 0.5mm; for thin slices, thick slices, strips and large pieces, the deviation should be less than 1mm; for the segments, less than 2mm.

（2）Size of Granules

After being purified, some drugs have to be ground by hand or machine into granules with different sizes to meet the special needs in clinic or to maintain the active ingredients, or just because they can't be sliced to pieces. The granules of the same kind should be even and clean. The classification on powder should follow the rules of *Chinese Pharmacopoeia*.

3. Color and Luster

In general, raw materials have their own color and luster, which may be changed during processing. For example, the color of drugs from flowers and leaves will fade after being sunburned, exposed and stored for a long time. The cross section of the raw pieces of Radix Astragali (*Huangqi*) show radial striations while the color of processed ones is always deeper. The pieces of raw Radix Glycyrrhizae (*Gancao*) are yellow, but the processed ones with honey become dark yellow. The processed Radix Rehmanniae (*Dihuang*) has black light comparing to the yellow color of raw pieces. The softening and cutting process can also influence the color and luster. For example, the color of Radix Scutellariae (*Huangqin*) will become green after being soaked in cold water.

According to *General Quality Standards*, besides the standards for different processed products in color and luster, all the processed ones should also obey the following rules. First, the color and luster should be even. Then, in the products processed with rice and liquid adjuvant materials (wine, vinegar, salt water, etc.), the content of the raw and burnt pieces should be less than 2%; in the scorched products, the content should be less than 3%; and in the products stir – fried into charcoal, the content of the raw pieces and the incinerated pieces should be less than 5%.

4. Odor

Both the raw materials and processed products have their own odor. Most Chinese herbal medicine, such as Radix Angelicae Sinensis (*Danggui*) and Herba Menthae (*Bohe*), which contain volatile oils, have strong fragrance. The terrible odor of some animal medicines, such as Bombyx batryticatus (*Jiangcan*) and Agkistrodon (*Qishe*), should be removed through processing. The processed products should have not only the original odor of themselves but also special odor of adjuvant materials, such as the odors of wine, vinegar, salt water, ginger juice and honey, etc.

5. Moisture Content

The moisture content is a basic index in quality control of the raw materials and processed products. Too much moisture content in the processed products will cause molds and damages by insect, but too less moisture content is also the reason for cracking of jel products.

Generally, the moisture content in the processed products should be controlled between 7% to 13%. According to *General Quality Standards*, the moisture content in the products stir – fried with honey should be less than 15%; in the products stir – fried with wine, vinegar, salt water and ginger juice, and steamed, boiled, fermented or germinated products, it should be less than 13%.

6. Ash Content

The content of physiological ash and acid – insoluble ash is an important index of purity detection in the processed products. The content of acid – insoluble ash in the same drug should be within a certain range. Too high content of physiological ash and acid – insoluble ash in the raw and processed products indicates that they have been mixed with some impurities like silt or mud. Generally, the content of ash in the products processed with adjuvant materials is higher than that in the raw materials.

7. Extractum

Both waster – soluble extracts and alcohol – soluble extracts can be used to evaluate the quality of the processed products. The extractum of the processed products, such as Rhizoma Corydalis (*Yanhusuo*) stir – fried with vinegar and Carapax et Plastrum Testudinis (*Guijia*) fired with sand, is often higher than that of the raw materials.

8. Active Ingredients

The quantity of active ingredient is the most reliable and accurate index for quality control in TCM. The amount and quality of some ingredients, such as alkaloid, glycosides and volatile oil, will change when the raw materials being processed. Therefore, to control the quality of processed products, the detection methods and the measurement standard should be established.

9. Toxic Ingredients

For the processed products with toxic ingredients, a limit is essential to guarantee the safety of clinical treatment. According to *Chinese Pharmacopoeia*, the total quantity of aconitine, hypaconitine and mesaconitine in Radix Aconiti Cocta (*Zhichuangwu*) should be less than 0. 04%, the content of fatty oil in processed Fructus Crotonis (*Badou*) should be 18. 0% ~20. 0%, and the content of strychnine in processed Semen Strychni (*Maqianzi*) should be 0. 78% ~0. 82%.

10. Hazardous Materials

The content of hazardous materials in processed products should also be limited to guarantee the safety of clinical treatment. Such materials include heavy metal, arsenic salt, residue of pesticide and so on. The processing could make the content of such hazardous materials lower than unprocessed ones.

11. Hygienic Inspection

Hygienic inspection is very essential to the quality control because drugs are easily contaminated during the production, processing, storage and transportation. In general, detection should be done with pathogenic bacteria, colibacillus, total number of bacteria and mold, living mites, fungus, aspergillus flavus and so on.

12. Packaging Inspection

The requirements of packaging should be in accordance with the provisions in *Drug Administration Law* and *Regulations for Implementation of the Drug Administration Law of the People's Republic of China*. The tag on the outside container must indicate the name, place of production, production date, certification of fitness, etc. Inside the individual packaging materials, the label should indicate all the above items, along with manufacturer and production batch number.

Section Two Storage

1. Storage History of Chinese Materia Medica Processing Products

The history of storage for the processed products can be divided into three periods, namely, traditional period, chemical period and period of modern techniques.

In the first period (from the Spring – autumn and Warring states to the Qing dynasty), storing methods include ventilating, solarization, baking, moisture absorption, sealing, and antagonism.

In the second period (from 1930's to 1970's), the chemical fumigants are often adopted.

In modern times (after 1980's), storing methods include air – conditioning maintenance storing technique, low temperature storage, etc.

2. Variation in Storage

(1) Mildewing and Rotting

When the drugs are exposed to moisture, fungus will grow in the form of hyphae over the surface under certain temperature. Heat, humidity and nutrients content of the processed products are the main causes of the breeding of fungus. Mildewing will destroy the active ingredient in the drug, or even generate toxicity, which will make the drug useless.

(2) Rotting due to Insect Bite

Chinese medicine and its processed products are easy to be bitten by insects to become hollow or broken pieces. The excrement and secretion of insects will also contaminate the medicine. The damages by the insects will cause mildewing, change of color and odor, rot, which will break down the active ingredient or even generate toxicity. In traditional methods of storage, when the temperature reaches 16℃ ~ 35℃, the relative humidity is above 70% and the moisture content is over 13%, there will become the best breeding ground for insects.

(3) Discoloration

Discoloration is the change in color of the medicine. Under certain conditions, the original color of the medicine can be changed or even disappear. These changes will not only bring problems in identifying but also indicate the decline in quality.

Discoloration is often caused by the instability or the reactions of some chemical composition, such as oxygenization, polymerization and hydrolyzation of enzyme. Improper methods of storage are another reason for the change of color. The color of some medicines, such as Radix Angelicae Dahuricae (*Baizhi*), Rhizoma Alismatis (*Zexie*), Radix Trichosanthis (*Tianhuafen*) and Rhizoma Dioscoreae (*Shanyao*), can be changed from light to deep, while for the medicines like Radix Astragali (*Huangqi*) and Cortex Phellodendri Chinensis (*Huangbo*), it is from deep to light. The color of flowers and leaves can be changed from bright to pale, such as Flos Lonicerae (*Jinyinhua*), Flos Chrysanthemi (*Juhua*), Folium Isatidis (*Daqingye*) and Folium Nelumbinis (*Heye*).

(4) Extensive Diffusion of Oil

Under certain temperature and humidity, the medicines that contain volatile oil, sugar and fat will have oil overflowing on the surface, become soft and tacky, and then go rancid. These are the symptoms of extensive diffusion of oil.

Under the high temperature environment, the unsaturated fatty acid in the grease medicine is often oxidized and decomposed to compounds of aldehyde and ketone, which makes the medicine go rancid. Such drugs include Semen Armeniacae Amarum (*Kuxingren*), Semen Persicae (*Taoren*), Semen Platycladi (*Baiziren*), Semen Pruni (*Yuliren*), fried Semen Raphani (*Laifuzi*), fried Semen Ziziphi Spinosae (*Suanzaoren*), Radix Angelicae Sinensis (*Danggui*), Cortex Cinnamomi (*Rougui*), Gekko *japonicus* Dumeril et Bibron (*Bihu*), Aspongopus (*Jiuxiangchong*), Corium Erinacei (*Ciweipi*), etc.

Drugs containing sugar may also have this phenomenon which is called sugar overflowing. Such drugs include Radix Asparagi (*Tiandong*), Radix Ophiopogonis (*Maidong*), Rhizoma Polygonati Odorati (*Yuzhu*), Radix Achyranthis Bidentatae (*Niuxi*), Rhizoma Polygonati (*Huangjing*) and Radix Rehmanniae Praeparata (*Shudihuang*).

(5) Efflorescence

Efflorescence is the loss of water of crystallization in mineral drugs when exposed to air or put in sufficiently dry environment. The change of the constituent structure will influence the quality and property. This often happens to the drugs like Natrii Sulfas (*Mangxiao*).

(6) Deliquesce

Deliquesce is the process in which some solid drugs that contain salt absorb moisture from the atmosphere until it dissolves and forms solution on the surface. This occurs easily to the drugs like Sal Praeparatum (*Xianqiushi*), Sal Ammoniac (*Naosha*), Halitum (*Daqingyan*) and Natrii Sulfas (*Mangxiao*). Therefore, these drugs are difficult to be stored.

(7) Adhesion

With moisture or heat, some drugs that contain hard resin or animal glue with low fusing point are easily adhering into clumps. Such drugs include Olibanum (*Ruxiang*), Myrrha (*Moyao*), Resina Ferulae (*Awei*), Aloe (*Luhui*), Catechu (*Ercha*), Colla Corii Asini (*E'jiao*), Cornu Cervi Pantotrichum (*Lujiaojiao*) and Chiemys Reevesii (*Guibanjiao*), etc.

(8) Volatilization

Volatilization is the loss of volatile oil in some drugs, which result in shriveling or breaking of the drugs. Exposure to the air, temperature and long time storage are the main causes for volatilization. Such drugs include Cortex Cinnamomi (*Rougui*), Lignum Aquilariae Resinatum (*Chenxiang*) and Cortex Magnoliae Officinalis (*Houpo*).

(9) Rottenness

Influenced by the temperature, air and microbes, some fresh drugs are easy to go rancid. Such drugs include fresh Radix Rehmanniae (*Dihuang*), fresh Rhizoma Zingiberis Recens (*Shengjiang*), fresh Rhizoma Phragmitis (*Lugen*), fresh Herba Dendrobii (*Shihu*), fresh Rhizoma Imperatae (*Maogen*), Rhizoma Acori Tatarinowii (*Shichangpu*) and so on. The rotten drugs cannot be used any more.

(10) Spontaneous Combustion

Some herbs, such as Flos Carthami (*Honghua*), Folinum Artemisiae Argyi (*Aiye*) and Radix et Rhizoma Nardostachyos (*Gansong*), are loose in texture. Improper drying before being stacked make the heat coming from bacterial metabolism unable to be released timely. When the temperature reaches over 67℃, the heat will lead to smoke or even fire. Then, there is no guarantee for quality of the drugs. Semen Platycladi (*Baiziren*) also has this problem.

3. Causes of the Variation

Many factors can lead to anomalies during the storage. These factors can be classified into two categories, internal factors (chemical compounds and moisture content) and external factors (origin, environment, biological and time). And the latter is usually the main cause.

(1) Internal Factors

①Moisture content: Moisture content is one of main factors that lead to anomalies during the storage. After being processed with water or other liquid adjuvant materials, drugs become easily damaged by insects, molds or become discolored. Then the active ingredients in drugs may dissolve in water or be broken down by hydrolysis or enzymolysis.

②Chemical composition: High content of nutrient in drugs is another cause to anomalies. For example, too much volatile oil will lead to the change of odor, release of oil or volatilization. High content of alkaloid sometimes leads to deterioration or discoloration.

(2) External Factors

①Environment

Sunlight: sunlight can fade or change the color of the drug, dissipate its fragrance and make it go rancid.

Air: the oxidation and ozone in the air make drugs containing volatile oil, fatty oil and saccharides easy to go rancid.

Temperature: the proper temperature for storage should be between 20℃ and 35℃.

Humidity: the proper relative humidity for storage should be between 60% and 70%.

②Biological factors: Biological factors here refer to the living things that will influence the quality of the drugs such as microbe, insects, hamster, birds, snakes, etc. Among them, microbe and insects are the main problems.

③Time：Long – term storage will reduce the active ingredient in drugs，leading to reduction even loss of drugs' effects. For example，after being stored for one year，the content of amygdalase in raw Semen Armeniacae Amarum (*Kuxingren*) and processed almonds will reduce from 4. 95% to 4. 37% and 4. 18% to 3. 66% respectively.

4. Methods for Storage

(1) Traditional Methods

When storing drugs with traditional methods，we should first keep the raw materials，processed products，store house and surrounding areas clean. Regular sterilizing is also necessary. And then，four kinds of methods are often used.

First，keep ventilation to help drying the drug in shade or sunshine.

Second，absorb moisture by using quick lime，charcoal，bamboo charcoal，plant ash，calcium chloride or silica gel.

Third，seal the container of the drug to prevent it from air，moisture，microorganism and pests.

Forth，combine more than two drugs together in storage or store the drug with materials with special odor. This kind of combination can prevent the drugs from molding or damaging due to insect bites. Such combination includes Flos Carthami (*Zanghonghua*) with Cordyceps (*Dongchongxiacao*)，Allii Sativi Bulbus (*Dasuan*) with Semen Euryales (*Qianshi*)，or Borneolum Syntheticum (*Bingpian*) with Medulla Junci (*Dengxincao*).

(2) Chemical Methods (fumigation)

Fumigation is a method of insect and bacterium control by using volatile chemicals such as sulfur dioxide，chloropicrin and aluminium phosphide (AlP) .

Sulfur dioxide (also sulfurous anhydride) is a toxic gas with irritating smell and can dissolve easily in water. When it is used in storing drugs，this chemical will destroy some active ingredients of the drug. And in order to minimize the residual of sulfur dioxide，arsenic，and mercury，sulphur dioxide should not be used in storing herbal medicines.

Chloropicrin is a toxic liquid which is severely irritating to the mucous membrane of eyes. But it is a good insecticide that can kill common insect in storehouse.

AlP also can be used to control insect and microbe.

(3) Modern Techniques

With the development of modern science，many new techniques have been used in storing. The wide application of these new storage methods makes drug storage more scientific and reasonable.

①Gas – regulating：Gas – regulating is often used to prevent the drugs from being damaged by insects and molds by reducing the oxygen content and increasing carbondioxide content.

②Moistureproof air curtain：Moistureproof air curtain is a device to prevent the cold air inside from leaking and hot – air outside invading.

③^{60}Co ray radiation: ^{60}Co ray radiation can be used to kill insects or microbe in the drugs.

④Storing at low temperature: Storing the drugs at low temperature can control the breeding of microbe and insect.

⑤Steam heating: There are three kinds of steam heating to disinfect the drug: LTLT (low temperature long time), HTST (high temperature short time) and UHT (ultra high temperature processing)

⑥Aseptic packaging: Aseptic packaging is to put the sterilized drugs in sterilized container.

⑦Dehumidifier: Dehumidifier is an appliance which reduces the level of humidity in the air.

⑧DMF (N, N – dimethyl formamide): DMF can inhibit the breeding of more than 30 kinds of molds, saccharomycetes and germ, especially aspergillus flavus.

⑨Desiccation and sterilization: The methods include far – infrared radiation and microwave sterilization.

⑩Pyrethrum insecticide: Pyrethrin is the active component of insecticide, it is the safest and the most effective natural insecticide.

⑪Stifling volatile oil: Volatile oil can be used to control the above – mentioned anomalies in herbal medicines.

All in all, the electrical control system should be applied in storehouse for real time monitoring. Keep an eye on the temperature and relative humidity regularly to make sure that they are under 25℃ and around 75%.

第五章 炮制品的质量要求及贮藏保管

第一节 炮制品的质量要求

1. 净度

（1）定义

净度可以用炮制品含杂质及非药用部位的限度来表示。

（2）具体要求

国家中医药管理局关于《中药饮片质量标准通则（试行）》的通知中规定，中药炮制品即中药饮片的净度要求是：不应该含有泥沙、灰屑、霉烂品、虫蛀品、杂物及非药用部位等。果实种子类、全草类、树脂类含药屑、杂质不得过3%；根类、根茎类、叶类、花类、藤木类、皮类、动物类、矿物类及菌藻类等含药屑、杂质不得过2%；炒制品（炒黄、米炒）、炙品（酒、醋、盐）、发酵制品、发芽制品含药屑、杂质不得过1%。

2. 片型及破碎度

（1）片型

片型的外观形状要符合《中国药典》（一部）及《全国中药炮制规范》的规定。切制后的饮片应均匀、整齐，色泽鲜明，表面光洁，无污染，无泛油等。《中药饮片质量标准通则（试行）》规定：异形片不得超过10%；极薄片不得超过该片标准厚度0.5mm；薄片、厚片、丝、块不得超过该片标准厚度1mm；段不得超过该标准厚度2mm。

（2）破碎度

一些药物不宜切制饮片，或有临床上的特殊需要，或为了更好地保留有效成分，可经净制处理后，用手工或机器直接破碎成不同规格的颗粒。这种颗粒应粒度均匀，无杂质，粉末的分等应符合《中国药典》的要求。

3. 色泽

中药饮片都有固定的颜色光泽与气味。生品有其固有的色泽，如花类药材和叶类药材因日晒或暴露过久，或贮存过久会导致其颜色退去。黄芪经切制后表面有菊花心，经炮制后颜色比原来加深；甘草生品黄色，蜜炙以后则变为老黄色；熟地黄则以乌黑光亮者为佳。药材软化切制的过程也会影响饮片的色泽，如黄芩冷浸后变绿。

关于炮制品的色泽要求，《中药饮片质量标准通则（试行）》规定，除应符合该品种的标准外，各炮制品的色泽要均匀。炒黄品、加辅料（酒、醋、盐等）炙品含生片、糊片不得超过2%；炒焦品含生片、糊片不得超过3%；炒炭品含生片和完全炭化者不得超过5%。

4. 气味

中药及其炮制品均有其固有的气味。大多数含有挥发油类中药都有浓烈的香气，如当归、薄荷；有些有不良气味的中药须用炮制的方法除去异味，如动物类药材僵蚕、蕲蛇；有些加辅料炙的药材，炙后除了具有原来药物的气味外，还具有辅料的气味，如酒炙、醋炙、盐炙、姜炙、蜜炙等。

5. 水分

水分是控制中药材及其炮制品质量的一个基本指标。炮制品中含水过多时容易造成发霉变质、虫蛀等，胶类药材含水少时可造成干裂，而成碎块。

一般炮制品的水分含量宜控制在7%～13%，各类炮制品的含水量，《中药饮片质量标准通则（试行）》中规定：蜜炙品不得超过15%；酒炙品、醋炙品、盐炙品、姜汁炙品、蒸制品、煮制品、发芽制品、发酵制品均不得超过13%。

6. 灰分

生理灰分与酸不溶性灰分是检测中药炮制品纯净度的重要指标，同种药物的酸不溶性灰分通常在一定范围之内。如果中药生品或炮制品中生理灰分或酸不溶性灰分含量过高，多数是混入泥沙等杂质。经过辅料炮制之后中药的灰分含量通常要高于原药材。

7. 浸出物

水溶性浸出物与醇溶性浸出物可用来衡量炮制品的质量，炮制品的浸出物质量通常要高于生品，如醋炙延胡索和砂烫龟甲。

8. 有效成分

有效成分的含量是控制中药质量的首选方法。中药炮制后其有效成分有的发生了量变，有的发生了质变，例如生物碱、苷类、挥发油等。应制定中药炮制品有效成分的检测方法及含量标准以控制炮制质量。

9. 有毒成分

为了确保中医临床用药安全有效，必须建立中药炮制品中所含有毒成分的含量限度。《中国药典》规定：制川乌含酯型生物碱以乌头碱、次乌头碱及新乌头碱的总量计，不得超过0.04%，巴豆的炮制品巴豆霜含脂肪油应为18%～20%，马钱子炮制品中含士的宁应为0.78%～0.82%。

10. 有害物质

为了确保中医临床用药安全有效，必须建立中药炮制品中所含有害物质的含量限度。

中药材中有害物质主要是指重金属、砷盐及残留的农药，通过炮制可使这类有害物质残留量降低。

11. 卫生学检查

中药材及饮片在生产、加工、储存、运输过程中易受杂菌污染，为保证其质量必须进行卫生学检查。检测内容主要有致病菌、大肠杆菌、细菌总数、霉菌总数、活螨、真菌及黄曲霉菌等。

12. 包装检查

中药饮片的包装必须符合《药品管理法》和《中华人民共和国药品管理法实施条例》规定，药品包装必须标明饮片名称、产地、生产日期、质量合格证等。饮片包装内的标签必须标明饮片名称、规格、产地、厂家、生产批号以及生产日期。

第二节　中药炮制品的贮藏保管

1. 中药炮制品贮存的发展

中药炮制品贮存的发展大致可分为 3 个时期，即传统时期、化学时期和现代技术时期。

传统时期（从春秋战国到清代以前），主要有通风、晾晒、烘烤、吸湿、密封、对抗等方法。

化学时期（从 20 世纪 30 年代到 70 年代），用化学熏蒸剂。

现代技术时代（20 世纪 80 年代以后），用气调养护、冷藏等。

2. 中药炮制品贮藏中的变异现象

（1）发霉

发霉是指药物受潮后，在适宜的温度下造成霉菌的滋生和繁殖，在药物表面布满菌丝的现象。高温、潮湿的贮存环境以及药材本身的营养物质是造成细菌滋生和繁殖的主要原因。发霉会破坏药材中有效成分的含量甚至产生毒性，最终导致不堪药用。

（2）虫蛀

虫蛀是指中药及其炮制品被仓虫啃噬，使药物被蛀空或蛀成碎片粉末的现象，另外，害虫蛀蚀药材或饮片时的排泄物和分泌物均可污染药物。虫蛀可引起中药及其炮制品发霉、变色、变味、腐烂，使中药的有效成分降低甚至产生毒性。传统法贮存中药在一定的温度和湿度环境下易引发虫蛀，一般而言，在环境温度 16℃ ~ 35℃，相对湿度大于 70%，药材本身含水量高于 13% 的条件下最容易引起仓虫繁殖。

（3）变色

变色是指药物的固有颜色发生了变化，或变为其他颜色，或失去原来颜色。颜色的变化既可造成外观的混乱，也可造成药品质量下降。

药物的化学成分不稳定或发生反应会使药物的颜色发生改变，如酶的氧化、聚合、水解反应。由于保管不当，常使某些药物的颜色由浅变深，或由白色变为黄色，如白芷、泽泻、天花粉、山药等；或由深变浅，如黄芪、黄柏等；或由鲜艳变黯淡，如花类的金银花、菊花等，叶类的大青叶、荷叶等。

（4）泛油

泛油是指含有挥发油、糖类和脂肪的药物，在一定温度、湿度的环境下，造成油脂外溢，质地返软、发黏，并发出油败气味的现象。

含油脂类药物在高温的环境中，其所含不饱和脂肪酸氧化、分解成醛、酮类化合物，出现酸败气味，如苦杏仁、桃仁、柏子仁、郁李仁、炒莱菔子、炒酸枣仁、当归、肉桂、壁虎、九香虫、刺猬皮等。

含糖类药材或饮片也会出现类似泛油的现象，而称"泛糖"，如天冬、麦冬、玉竹、牛膝、黄精、熟地等。

（5）风化

风化是指某些含有结晶水的矿物药，经风吹日晒或过分干燥而逐渐失去结晶水成为粉末的现象。药物的组成结构发生改变，也影响到药物的质量和功效，如芒硝极易风化失水。

（6）潮解

潮解是指某些盐类固体药物容易吸收潮湿空气中的水分，使其表面慢慢溶化成液体状态，如咸秋石、硇砂、大青盐、芒硝等。易潮解的药物相对难于贮存。

（7）粘连

粘连是指某些熔点比较低的固体树脂类或动物胶类药物，受潮、吸热后容易黏结成块，如乳香、没药、阿魏、芦荟、儿茶、阿胶、鹿角胶、龟板胶等。

（8）挥发

某些含挥发油的药物，因受空气和温度以及贮存日久的影响，使挥发油散失，失去油润，产生干枯或破裂的现象，如肉桂、沉香、厚朴等。

（9）腐烂

腐烂是指某些鲜活药物，因受温度、空气及微生物的影响，使微生物的繁殖和活动增加，导致药物酸败、腐臭，如鲜生地、鲜生姜、鲜芦根、鲜石斛、鲜茅根、鲜菖蒲等。药物一旦腐烂即不可使用。

（10）冲烧

冲烧又叫自燃，质地轻薄松散的植物药材，如红花、艾叶、甘松等，由于本身干燥不适度，或在包装码垛前吸潮，在紧实状态中细菌代谢产生的热量不能散发，当温度积聚到67℃以上时，热量便能从中心一下冲到垛外，轻者起烟，重者起火，药材质量也就不复保证了。柏子仁也容易产生自燃现象。

3. 中药炮制品变异的原因

中药炮制品在贮存过程中会发生很多变异现象，究其原因总的来说有两个方面。一是炮制品本身的性质（化学成分和含水量），二是炮制品贮存的外界条件（基原因素、环境因素、生物因素、时间因素），影响炮制品变异的主要原因是外部因素。

（1）自身性质

①含水量：水分是导致药物在贮存过程中出现变异的主要原因之一。药材经过水或液

体辅料处理后易发生虫蛀、发霉、变色等变异现象，使有效成分溶于水，或发生水解、酶解反应而降低有效成分含量。

②化学成分：营养物质含量高易导致变异，挥发油含量高易导致变味、走油或挥发，生物碱类成分含量高易造成变质和变色。

（2）外部因素

①环境因素

日光：可使药材颜色渐褪或变色，使具香气中药的气味散失，使含油脂类饮片酸败。

空气：空气中的氧气和臭氧可使含挥发油、脂肪油、糖类成分的药物产生变异。

温度：一般药物在 20℃ ~35℃时比较稳定。

湿度：一般炮制品相对湿度要在 60% ~70%。

②生物因素：生物因素主要包括微生物、仓虫、仓鼠以及鸟类、蛇类等，其中最主要的是微生物和仓虫。

③时间因素：长期贮存会造成有效成分的降低，从而使药物降低甚至失去疗效，如苦杏仁放置一年之后，其中苦杏仁酶的含量由 4.95% 降至 4.37%，其炮制品含量则从 4.18% 降至 3.66%。

4. 贮藏保管方法

（1）传统贮藏保管方法

要保持中药材及其炮制品、仓库以及周边环境的清洁卫生，并对仓库进行消毒。

①通风：可将药物阴干或晒干。

②吸湿：可使用生石灰、木炭、竹炭、草木灰、氯化钙、硅胶等。

③密封：是隔绝空气、湿气、微生物、害虫的一种贮存方法。

④对抗：将两种或两种以上的药物放在一起保存，或将药物与具有特殊气味的物质同贮，以防止霉变或虫蛀的一种贮存方法。如藏红花和冬虫夏草同贮，大蒜和芡实同贮，冰片和灯心草同贮。

（2）化学熏蒸法

化学熏蒸法是一种使用挥发性化学物质进行杀虫灭菌的方法，如二氧化硫、氯化苦、磷化铝。

二氧化硫，又称亚硫酸酐，具有强烈的刺激性，在水中溶解度大。但是二氧化硫会破坏一些药材的有效成分，为了避免诸如二氧化硫、砷、汞等有害物质的残留，植物类中药材的贮藏应避免使用二氧化硫。

氯化苦，对眼睛黏膜有很强的刺激作用，并且杀虫力强，能杀灭常见的害虫。

磷化铝，杀虫力强，并可抑制和杀灭微生物。

（3）现代贮存保管方法

随着现代科技的不断发展，中药的贮藏保管引入越来越多的新技术，这些新型贮藏方法的广泛应用，使得中药贮藏保管更加科学化和合理化。

①气调养护：通过降低氧气含量加入二氧化碳以达到杀虫防霉的作用。

②气幕防潮：是一种防止库内冷空气派出库外、库外潮湿空气侵入库内的装置。

③钴-60 射线辐射：钴-60 射线可杀死附着于药物的虫类和微生物。

④低温冷藏：利用低温抑制微生物和仓虫的滋生和繁殖。

⑤蒸汽加热：可分为低高温长时间灭菌、亚高温短时间灭菌、超高温瞬时灭菌三种方法。

⑥无菌包装：中药材、饮片或其炮制品灭菌后装入一个霉菌、杂菌无法生长的容器内的方法。

⑦除湿机：利用空气除湿机吸收空气中的水分以降低相对湿度。

⑧二甲基甲酰胺：二甲基甲酰胺可抑制 30 余种霉菌、酵母菌和细菌，尤其可抑制黄曲霉的滋生。

⑨干燥和灭菌：主要有远红外辐射灭菌法和微波杀菌法。

⑩除虫菊杀虫剂：除虫菊酯是杀虫剂的有效活性成分，是一种最为安全有效的天然杀虫剂。

⑪挥发油抑制法：利用挥发油的挥发来抑制植物类中药材及其炮制品的变异。

总之，贮藏中药饮片或其炮制品的库房中要建立电子操控设备，随时检查库内情况，保持库内温度在 25℃以下，相对湿度 75% 左右。

Chapter Six   Cleansing

Section One   The Purpose of Cleansing

Cleansing is the first working procedure of processing raw Chinese medicines. There may be sand mixed in drugs during collection, and the drugs may mildew and rot, or rot due to insect bites in storage. What's more, during the processing, medicinal parts need to be picked out, and non – medicinal parts need to be removed.

Cleansing is a working process of selecting medicinal parts and removing non – medicinal parts, impurities and mildewed materials to satisfy the purity criteria before cutting, processing and compounding the drug.

The purposes of cleansing include separating different medicinal parts, classifying drugs according to size and thickness, removing non – medicinal parts and impurities.

Section Two   Removing Impurities

There are many ways to remove impurities. As each way is applicable to different drugs, the proper way should be chosen with flexibility according to the actual situation. These ways are sorting, screening, selection in wind and selection in water, etc.

1. Sorting

Sorting is to remove impurities and mildewed and rotten materials from the drug, or classify drugs according to size and thickness.

Operation methods: Put the raw drugs in long bamboo plaque or on the table, then pick out the useless impurities that cannot be sifted, such as nucleus, stem, moth – eaten damages, and mildewed and rotten parts, etc.

2. Screening

Screening is to sift out sand and impurities by using different sifters according to the shapes and sizes of drugs and impurities. Sands and impurities are sifted out to keep the drugs clean, such as bamboo sifter, iron sifter, tortoise plastron sifter, and net sifter, etc.

Mechanical sifters are now often used, such as oscillating type machine for sieving and micro motor – driven sifter. The latter is suitable for toxical and irritant drugs as well as drugs which are easily efflorescenced and deliquesced.

3. Selection in Wind

It means separating impurities from drugs by wind according to different weights of impurities and drugs. This way is usually suitable for drugs whose non – medicinal part, such as carpopodium, pedicel or shriveled parts, could be removed by wind.

4. Selection in Water

It refers to the method that selecting or removing impurities such as sands, salt or dirt through filtering or rinsing drugs. According to the different characters of drugs, methods of selection in water include washing, rinsing and immersing.

Washing is the way of washing drugs in bamboo baskets, then rinsing away the impurities such as earth, dust or mouldy spots.

Rinsing refers to rinsing drugs in a small container with much water to remove earth and sand or other impurities on the surface of the drug.

Immersing means soaking drugs in the container with much water for a long time, then turning over the drugs properly and changing water every day to decrease the toxin, salt and bad odor of the drugs.

There are some other ways of cleansing, such as picking, rubbing, wiping, milling, brushing, cutting with scissors or knife, digging and peeling, etc.

Section Three　Removing and Separating Different Medicinal Parts

According to the situation of raw drugs and clinical treatment requirement, different medicinal parts, such as remnant root or stem, bark or testa, hair, pith of plant, residual parts of stem, nucleus, pulp, head, tail, foot and wing, remnant meat, impurities, mould materials, etc. needed to be removed or separated.

1. Removing Remnant Root or Stem

Generally speaking, removing remnant root is to remove the non – medicinal roots of herbs, such as taproot, rootlet, fibrous root, etc. It is often used in Herba Schizonepetae (*Jingjie*), Herba Ephedrae (*Mahuang*), Rhizoma Coptidis (*Huanglian*), etc.

Removing remnant stem is to remove non – medicinal stems of herbs. It is used in Radix Gentianae (*Longdancao*), Radix Salviae Miltiorrhizae (*Danshen*), Radix Dipsaci (*Xuduan*), etc.

If the same kind of drug's root and stem with different effects can both be used, they must be separated. For example, the root and stem of Herba Ephedrae (*Mahuang*) need to be separated because its root has the effect of hidroschesis but its stem has the effect of diaphoresis.

Working methods: remove non – medicinal parts by cutting with scissors, rubbing, selecting in wind or sorting, etc.

2. Removing Stalk

It refers to remove the non – medicinal parts of fruits, flowers and leaves to make the dose accurate, such as removing old stem or the base of flower or fruit. It is suitable for Fructus Schisandrae (*Wuweizi*), Magnolia liliflora (*Mulan*), Fructus Gardeniae (*Zhizi*), etc.

Working methods: remove the non – medicinal parts by selecting, cutting and picking, etc.

3. Removing Bark or Testa

Removing bark means removing the cork, velamen, fruit peel or testa of drugs. It is done to facilitate cutting drugs into pieces, making the dose accurate, separating different medicinal parts and discarding the non – medicinal parts.

Cork, moss and other dirty things can be removed from bark drugs by scarping barks, such as Cortex Magnoliae Officinalis (*Houpo*), Cortex Phellodendri Chinensis (*Huangbo*) and Cortex Eucommiae (*Duzhong*) with knife. Barks needs to be removed from trees in their habitats when they are still fresh, such as Rhizoma Anemarrhenae (*Zhimu*) and Radix Platycodi (*Jiegeng*). Peel or testa need to be removed from some fruit or seed drugs by crushing or scalding, such as Fructus Tsaoko (*Caoguo*), Fructus Amomi (*Sharen*).

4. Removing Fine Hair

It means removing fine hair, squama on the drug's surface and fibrous root to avoid irritation such as cough or any other side – effects, and to make drugs cleaner.

Fine hair needs to be cleared from some rhizome drugs by heating with sand or striking, such as Rhizoma Drynariae (*Gusuibu*), Rhizoma Cyperi (*Xiangfu*), and Rhizoma Anemarrhenae (*Zhimu*).

Fine hair can be removed from some leaf drugs by brushing with coir brush, such as Folium Eriobotryae (*Pipaye*) and Folium Pyrrosiae (*Shiwei*).

There is flaxen tomenta in the inner side of the seeds of Fructus Rosae Laevigatae (*Jinyingzi*), so hand tools are often used to dig out the fine hair and nucleus.

For other drugs, such as Cornu Cervi Pantotrichum (*Lurong*), the outside hair needs to be scrapped with ceramic chips or glass sheets. And then burn remnant hair in fire. Be careful not to burn the drug.

5. Discarding Pith of Plant

Pith of plant refers to hadromestome or embryonic germ of the drugs whose medicinal parts are roots and stems. Discarding pith of plant includes getting rid of the hadromestome and withered or rotten parts of the stems. For drugs whose medicinal parts are seeds, embryonic germs need to be discarded. Pith of plant needs to be removed from such drugs as Cortex Lycii (*Digupi*), Acanthopanax (*Wujiapi*), and Radix Morindae Officinalis (*Bajitian*).

The purposes of discarding pith of plant can be summed up into the following three aspects. The first is to remove the non – medicinal parts. Take Radix Morindae Officinalis (*Bajitian*) as an example, the proportion of hadromestome is higher and its effect is lower, which may influence the accuracy of the dose in clinic, so it needs to be discarded. The second is to separate the different medicinal parts. For example, nuts of Semen Nelumbinis (*Lianzi*) have the effect of clearing heart fire and relieving restlessness, and its pulp can nourish spleen and astringe sperm, they should be used respectively. The last is to eliminate side – effects, taking drugs without discarding the pith of plant will make patients feel suffocated, such as Radix Polygalae (*Yuanzhi*) .

6. Removing Nucleus

For some pulp drugs, the pulp instead of nucleus is often used as medicinal part. Some of these nucleus (or seeds) are non – medicinal parts, while some are medicinal parts, so different parts should be used respectively. Drugs of this kind include Fructus Corni (*Shanzhuyu*), Fructus Mume (*Wumei*), Fructus Crataegi (*Shanzha*), Fructus Chebulae (*Hezi*), etc. The purpose of removing nucleus is to prevent spermatorrhea in traditional thought. Modern studies believe that it is because nucleus has less effective components. In modern times, the purpose is thought to improve clinical efficiency, guarantee the accuracy of dispensing drugs and make the effective components easier to be decocted.

The methods of selection in wind, screening, sorting, immersion, cutting and digging are often used in removing nucleus.

7. Removing Residual Parts of Stem

Residual parts of stem refer to the residual parts of root, rootstalk, stem base, or phytyl group. The purpose is to avoid the vomitive side – effect in traditional thought. Modern studies have found that there is not any vomitive side – effect in the residual parts of Panax ginseng (*Renshen*), so it is unnecessary to discard residual parts of root of Panax ginseng (*Renshen*) .

8. Removing Pulp

Pulp must be removed from some fruit drugs before they are used in clinic, such as Fructus Aurantii Immaturus (*Zhishi*), Fructus Aurantii (*Zhiqiao*), Pericarpium Citri Reticulatae Viride (*Qingpi*), Fructus Chaenomelis (*Mugua*) . In traditional thought, the purpose of removing pulp is to avoid side – effect of flatulence. Modern studies believe that the purposes of removing pulp are to remove non – medicinal parts so as not to reduce the effect, avoid mildewing and rotting due to insect bite, as well as relieve bitter, sour and astringent tastes of drugs.

9. Removing Head, Tail, Skin, Bone, Foot and Wing

In order to get rid of toxical parts or non – medicinal parts, the head, tail, foot or wing needs to be removed from some animal or insect drugs. For example, head and tail must be removed from Agkistrodon (*Qishe*); head and feet must be removed from Scolopendra (*Wugong*); head, feet and wings must be removed from Mylabris (*Banmao*).

The methods of removing head, tail, skin and bone include immersing and then cutting, or steaming and then divesting. While the methods of discarding head, foot and wing are breaking off or picking with hands.

10. Removing Remnant Meat

In order to purify drugs, remnant meat and fascia must be removed from some animal drugs, such as Carapax et Plastrum Testudinis (*Guijia*), Carapax Trionycis (*Biejia*), bones of animals, etc. The traditional methods are to scrape by knife, pick or soak in some chemical reagent. Currently, pancreas enzymolysis and microzyme zymolysis are used to remove the remnant meat efficiently.

第六章 净选加工

第一节 净选加工的目的

净制是中药炮制第一道工序。药物在收集过程中会混有沙子，在储存过程中会发生霉变和虫蛀。药物也要选取规定的药用部位，除去非药用部位。

净制是在切制、炮炙或调配、制剂前，选取规定的药用部位，除去非药用部位、杂质及霉变品，使其达到药物纯度标准的方法。

净制的目的：

1. 分离药用部位。
2. 按照药物大小、粗细进行分档。
3. 除去非药用部位。
4. 除去杂质。

第二节 清除杂质

清除杂质的方法有许多种。每一种除杂方法都可以适用于多种药物，必须根据实际情况灵活的选用恰当的方法。根据方法的不同，可分为挑选、筛选、风选和水选等。

1. 挑选

挑选是清除混在药物中的杂质及霉变品等，或将药物按大小、粗细等进行分档。

操作方法：将药物放在竹长匾内或摊放在桌上，用手拣去簸不出、筛不下且不能入药的杂质，如核、梗或虫蛀、霉变等部分。

2. 筛选

筛选是根据药物和杂质的体积大小不同，选用不规格的筛和罗，以筛去药物中的砂石、杂质，使其达到洁净。筛有许多种，如竹筛、铁丝筛、龟板筛、网筛等。

现多用机械操作，主要有震荡式筛药机和小型电动筛药机。后者较适用于有毒、有刺激性及易风化、潮解的药物。

3. 风选

风选是利用药物和杂质的比重不同，借药材起伏的风力，使之与杂质分离的方法。此法主要适用于通过风选可将果柄、花梗、干瘪之物等非药用部位除去的药物。

4. 水选

水选是将药物通过水，将药物中附着的泥沙、盐分或不洁之物等杂质选出或漂去的方法。根据药材性质，水选可分为洗净、淘洗和浸漂。

洗净系将药物装在竹筐内，用清水将药材表面的泥土、灰尘、霉斑或其他不洁之物洗去。

淘洗是将药物置于小盛器内，用大量清水荡洗附在药物表面的泥沙或杂质。

浸漂是将药物置于大量清水中浸较长时间，适当翻动，每天换水，至药材毒质、盐分或腥臭异味得以减除为度。

此外，净制方法还有摘、揉、擦、碾、刷、剪切、挖、剥等。

第三节　清除和分离不同药用部位

根据原药材情况，结合中医临床用药要求，通过去根去茎，去皮壳，去毛，去心，去芦，去核，去瓤，去枝梗，去头尾足翅，去残肉，去杂质、霉变品等来清除和分离不同药用部位。

1. 去根去茎

去残根，一般指除去主根、支根、须根等非药用部位。常用于荆芥、麻黄、黄连等。

去残茎，一般指去除非药用部位的残茎，如龙胆草、丹参、续断等。

另外，同一类植物根、茎均能入药，但二者作用不同，须分离，分别入药。如麻黄根能止汗，茎能发汗解表，故须分开入药。

制作：一般采用剪切、搓揉、风选、挑选等。

2. 去枝梗

指除去某些果实、花、叶类药物非药用部位，如去除老茎枝、柄蒂，使用量准确。适用于五味子、木兰、栀子等药物。

制作：采用挑选、切除、摘等方法。

3. 去皮壳

药材去皮包括几个方面，有皮类药材去除其栓皮，根及根茎类药材去除其根皮，果实、种子类药材去除其果皮或种皮。去皮壳的目的主要有便于切片，使用量准确，分开药用部位，除去非药用部位等。

树皮类药物，如厚朴、黄柏、杜仲可用刀刮去栓皮、苔藓及其他不洁物。有些药物多在产地趁鲜去皮，如知母、桔梗等。果实或种子类药物，如草果、砂仁等可砸破皮壳，去壳取仁或可用燀法去皮。

4. 去毛

去毛是去掉药材表面的细绒毛、鳞片，以及根茎类药材的须根，以防服后刺激咽喉引起咳嗽或其他有害作用，并使药物清洁。

某些根茎类药材如骨碎补、香附、知母等表面具毛，需使用砂烫法或撞去绒毛的方法去毛。

部分叶类药材如枇杷叶、石韦等，须用棕刷刷去绒毛。

金樱子果实内部生有淡黄色绒毛，须用手工工具挖尽毛核。

其他药物如鹿茸，先用瓷片或玻璃片将其表面绒毛基本刮干净后，再用酒精燃着火将剩余的毛燎焦，注意不能将鹿茸燎焦。

5. 去心

"心"，指根茎药材的木质部或种子的胚芽。去心包括去根的木质部和枯朽部分、种子的胚等。地骨皮、五加皮、巴戟天等药材去心。

去心主要有三个目的。第一个目的是去除非药用部位，如巴戟天，由于木心所占比重较大，且无药效，影响用量的准确性，故要求去除。第二个目的是分离不同的药用部位。如莲子，莲子心能清心热、除烦，莲子肉能补脾涩精，故须分别入药。最后一个目的是消除药物的副作用。如远志不去心，服之会令人闷。

6. 去核

有些果肉类药物，常用果肉而不用核。其中有的核（或种子）属于非药用部位，有些属于药用部位，故须分别用药。如乌梅、山茱萸、山楂、诃子等。去核的目的可按传统的说法总结为的"去核者免滑精"。现代研究认为，去核是因为核中所含药效成分含量更低。到了近代，认为去核的目的是增强药效、保证用药准确以及利于药物有效成分的煎出。

去核制作时一般采用风选、筛选、挑选、浸润、切挖等方法。

7. 去芦

"芦"，指药物的根头、根茎、残茎、残基、叶基等部位。去芦传统的说法是"去芦者免吐"。现代研究未发现人参芦有催吐作用，认为人参没有必要去芦。

8. 去瓤

有些果实类药物，如枳实、枳壳、青皮、木瓜等，须去瓤用于临床。去瓤的目的，传统的说法是"去瓤者免胀"。现代研究认为，去瓤是为了去除非药用部位，以免降低药效，也可以防止药物霉变和虫蛀，又能降低药物的苦酸涩味。

9. 去头尾、皮骨、足、翅

部分动物类或昆虫类药物，为了除去有毒部位或非药用部位，需要去头尾或足翅。如蕲蛇须去头尾，蜈蚣须去头足，斑蝥须去头足翅。

去头尾、皮骨，一般采用浸润切除、蒸制剥除等方法。去头足翅，一般采用掰除、挑选等方法。

10. 去残肉

有些动物类药物，如龟甲、鳖甲、动物骨头等，须除去残肉筋膜，以纯净药物。传统的方法一般采用刀刮、挑选、用化学试剂浸漂等。现代可用胰脏净制法和酵母菌净制法。

Chapter Seven   Cutting of Prepared Drugs in Pieces

1. Definition of Prepared Drugs in Pieces

Generally speaking, any drugs used in traditional Chinese medicinal prescription or formulated medicine are called prepared drugs in pieces.

Narrowly speaking, prepared drugs in pieces refer to sliced drugs for Chinese medical prescription.

2. Definition of Cutting of Prepared Drugs in Pieces

Cutting of prepared drugs in pieces is a kind of processing technology of cutting drugs into specific slices, slivers, chops, sections, etc. after they are cleansed and softened.

3. Classification

The cutting methods can be divided into cutting by hand and cutting by machinery.

4. History

Cutting of prepared drugs in pieces originated from mouth – biting, which was recorded in *Formulas for Fifty – two Diseases* (*Wushierbingfang*) and *Canon of Medicine* (*Neijing*) .

5. Purpose

The purpose of cutting is to facilitate the decoction of the drugs' effective components, processing, preparation, identification and storage.

Section One   Processing with Water before Cutting

The purposes of processing with water before cutting are making drugs soften and easy to cut, moderating drugs' nature and reducing toxicity, cleaning drugs and discarding non – medicinal parts.

The principle of softening drugs is "less soaking, more moistening, penetrating drugs' interior with proper amount of water" . Some drugs should be cut in the habitats when they are fresh. Apart from soaking in water, there are some special methods for softening. For example, Radix Scutellariae

(*Huangqin*) should be softened by steaming; Colla Corii Asini (*E'jiao*) should be softened by baking.

1. Common Methods of Processing with Water

Common methods of processing with water include showering, elutriation (washing), soaking, rinsing, and moistening.

(1) Showering

Showering is to shower drugs with water. It is suitable for drugs with fragrant odor and drugs whose effective components are easy to lose with water, such as Herba Menthae (*Bohe*), Herba Schizonepetae (*Jingjie*), etc. The standard is the root becoming soft.

(2) Elutriation (washing)

Elutriation is a method of washing or fast lavation with clean water. It is suitable for soft – texture drugs whose effective components are easy to lose with water, such as Cortex Acanthopancis Radicis (*Wujiapi*), Radix Glycyrrhizae (*Gancao*), Semen Arecae (*Binglang*), etc. The standard is cleanness of drugs. Try to avoid using too much water. Currently, drug – washing machines are usually used.

(3) Soaking

Traditional method of soaking is suitable for scleroid drugs, such as Radix Aucklandiae (*Muxiang*), Radix Linderae (*Wuyao*) etc.

Fast soaking method is suitable for drugs whose texture is loose, soft and easy to get moist, such as Rhizoma seu Radix Notopterygii (*Qianghuo*); aromaticity drugs with essential oil and drugs full of phlegmatic temperament such as Radix Angelicae Sinensis (*Danggui*). The standard is complete softness of the drug.

When processing, immerse the drugs in water thoroughly. Immersing time should be as short as possible, depending on the quality of drugs, temperature of water, and seasons. Classify drugs according to size and remain some room for drug swelling after absorbing water.

(4) Rinsing

This method is suitable for toxic drugs, drugs pickled with salt and drugs with fishy smell, such as Radix Aconiti Lateralis Praeparata (*Fuzi*), Radix Aconiti (*Chuanwu*), Thallus Laminariae (*Haidai*), Placenta hominis (*Ziheche*) etc. The standard is the disappearance of irritating, salty taste and fishy smell.

(5) Moistening

This method is suitable for hard texture drugs. The methods are immersion, moistening with cover and moistening without cover.

Immersion is suitable for hard texture drugs, such as Rhizoma Coptidis (*Huanglian*), Radix Aucklandiae (*Muxiang*), etc.

Moistening with cover means covering drugs in a tight container to make them soften. It is also suitable for hard texture drugs, such as Radix Curcumae (*Yujin*), Rhizoma Chuanxiong (*Chuanxiong*).

Moistening without cover is suitable for drugs with carbohydrate or lipid, such as Radix Angelicae Sinensis (*Danggui*), Radix Scrophulariae (*Xuanshen*), Radix Achyranthis Bidentatae (*Niuxi*), *etc.* Steaming moistening and steam – spraying moistening can also be used.

There are two ways to improve softening by using machine. The feature of vacuum moistening method is to shorten time and avoid damaging the useful part. Diminution of pressure and cold soaking method can make water penetrate into the interior of the drug quickly and hence improve the efficiency of softening drugs.

2. Methods of Inspecting Softening Degree

（1）Bending

It is suitable for sliver type drugs, such as Radix Paeoniae Alba (*Baishao*) and Rhizoma Dioscoreae (*Shanyao*).

（2）Pinching with Finger

It is suitable for clumping type drugs, such as Rhizoma Atractylodis Macrocephalae (*Baizhu*), Radix Angelicae Dahuricae (*Baizhi*) and Rhizoma Alismatis (*Zexie*).

（3）Puncture

It is suitable for bulky type drugs, such as Radix et Rhizoma Rhei (*Dahuang*).

（4）Pinching with Hands

It is suitable for irregular type drugs.

（5）Splitting

It is suitable for large bulk and regular drugs.

Section Two   Types and Cutting Ways of Prepared Drugs in Pieces

1. Types

（1）Types and Sizes

Extremely thin slice 0. 5mm, such as Cornu Saigae Tataricae (*Lingyangjiao*).

Thin slice 1 ~ 2mm, such as Radix Paeoniae Alba (*Baishao*).

Thick slice 2 ~ 4mm, such as Poria (*Fuling*).

Oblique slice 2 ~ 4mm, such as Ramulus Cinnamomi (*Guizhi*), Radix et Rhizoma Rhei (*Dahuang*), Radix Glycyrrhizae (*Gancao*).

Straight slice 2 ~ 4mm, such as Radix Polygoni Multiflori (*Heshouwu*).

Sliver thin sliver 2 ~ 3mm, such as Cortex Phellodendri Chinensis (*Huangbo*) wide sliver. 5 ~ 10mm, such as Cortex Magnoliae Officinalis (*Houpo*).

Section 10 ~ 15mm, such as Herba Menthae (*Bohe*).

Chop 8 ~ 12mm^3 , such as Colla Corii Asini (*E'jiao*).

（2）Cutting Ways

The main ways of cutting include vertical cutting, cross cutting and titled cutting.

（3）Principles

According to their different medicinal parts, root and rhizome drugs should be cut into slices; and horny drugs should be cut into extremely thin slices or powder.

According to their different texture and shape, hard pykno – texture drugs should be cut into thin slices, while drugs of rarefaction and brittleness should be cut into thick slices; large and pykno – texture drugs should be cut into straight slices, while sliver shape drugs can be cut into oblique slices.

2. Cutting Methods of Prepared Drugs in Pieces

The methods of cutting include cutting by handwork, machinery and other methods.

（1）Handwork

It includes Machinery Mince knife and Rotation knife. There are some special tools, such as "clamp cutting" for Semen Arecae (*Binglang*) nut and processing kettle for Cornu Cervi Pantotrichum (*Lurong*).

（2）Machinery

There are Chopping Knife Cutting Machine, Rotary Cutting Machine and Multifunction Cutting Machine and so on.

Chopping Knife Cutting Machine is mainly applied to roots, rhizomes, whole plant herbs, not suitable for cutting granular drugs.

Rotary Cutting Machine generally applies to the class of grain – like drugs and clump herbs, not suitable for the whole plant drugs.

Multifunctional Cutting Machine is mainly applied to the roots, bulk herbs and fruits, and a variety of oblique prepared drugs in pieces.

（3）Other Methods

Pounding is suitable for horny drugs, such as Cornu Saigae Tataricae (*Lingyangjiao*).

Digging is suitable for xylon or horny drugs, such as Lignum Santali Albi (*Tanxiang*), Lignum Pini Nodi (*Songjie*), etc.

In addition, there are other cutting methods, including rasping, splitting, grinding, striking, etc.

Section Three   Dryness of Prepared Drugs in Pieces

1. Air Drying

（1）Features

Special equipments are not needed for air drying. And it is suitable for all types of prepared drugs in pieces, but limited by place and climate, and easy to be contaminated.

（2）Classifications

Drying in shade: It is suitable for drugs containing fragrant components, such as Herba Menthae (*Bohe*) and drugs with beautiful color. Flos Carthami (*Honghua*) is an example.

Drying in sunshine: It is suitable for viscidity drugs containing saccharic, such as Rhizoma Polygonati (*Huangjing*); powdery drugs, such as Rhizoma Dioscoreae (*Shanyao*); oiliness drugs, such as Radix Angelicae Sinensis (*Danggui*); color and luster drugs, such as Bulbus Fritillaria (*Beimu*).

2. Artificial Drying

（1）Features

The features of artificial drying are quick drying; not limited by place and climate; neat and clean; in need of equipments and energy.

（2）Equipment

They are mainly the inverted plate drying machine, hot air dryer, microwave drying technology and solar collector drying technology.

（3）Temperature

The temperature for normal drugs should be less than 80℃, while for drugs containing fragrant components, the temperature should be less than 50℃.

（4）Moisture Content

The moisture content of the prepared drug in pieces after drying should be between 7% and 13%.

（5）Notices

The notices include removing dampness in drying – room before drying, controlling time and temperature of drying, cooling the drugs after drying and making sure the moisture content after drying is between 7% and 13%.

Section Four　Packing of Prepared Drugs in Pieces

1. Functions

（1）It can facilitate storage, transportation, and selling.

（2）It helps to improve the drugs' sales and avoid drugs being contaminated again.

（3）It makes prepared drugs in pieces beautiful, clean and hygienic, and easy for regular supervision and inspection.

（4）It promotes modernization and standardization of the production of decoction pieces.

（5）It is beneficial for clinical prescriptions.

（6）It facilitates international trade of prepared drugs in pieces of TCM.

2. Notices of Packing

（1）Precious and toxic drugs are better to store in small glass bottles and paper boxes with instruction labels.

（2）Pay attention to decoration and ENA code of packing.

Section Five   Adverse Influences on the Quality of Prepared Drugs in Pieces

1. Failed Pieces

Failed pieces refer to all the pieces that don't meet the specification standards of cutting, including unbroken pieces, fringe or centre fallen pieces, wrinkle pieces, etc.

（1）Unbroken Pieces

They refer to unbroken pieces between adjacent intersections. It is due to too much water in the drugs when they are being softened or dull cutting knife.

（2）Fringe or Centre Fallen Pieces

They refer to the center part and fringe of pieces separated or broken. It is due to different hardness between different parts of the drugs after they are being softened.

（3）Wrinkle Pieces

They refer to rough sections with fish scales – like phenomenon. It is due to inadequate water when the drugs are being softened or dull cutting knife.

2. Curling Pieces

The fringes are curling and uneven showing on the surface of prepared drugs in pieces. It is due to too much water inside the drugs when they are being softened.

3. Allochromasia and Palling

It refers to the loss of luster and smell of the original drugs after they are dried. It is due to too long time of soaking or improper storing place for drying.

4. Extensive Diffusion of Oil

It refers to greasy surface or exuding mucus. It is due to too much water absorbed when the drugs are softened or too high temperature of the environment.

5. Mildewing

It refers to tiny fungus forming mycelium coating on the prepared drugs in pieces at appropriate temperature and in damp conditions.

Section Six   Other Processing Methods

1. Grinding

Grinding is suitable for minerals, such as Pyritum (*Zirantong*) and shell drugs like Squama Manis (*Chuanshanjia*), fruits and seeds, such as Fructus Gardeniae (*Zhizi*), small shape tuber, such as Bulbus Fritillaria (*Beimu*).

The purposes of grinding are to facilitate dissolution of effective components and make prescription and preparation easy.

2. Fine Hair Making

Herba Ephedrae (*Mahuang*) could be made into ephedrae fine hair to moderate its effects.

3. Mix with Adjuvant Materials

Indigo Naturalis (*Qingdai*) and Cinnabaris (*Zhusha*) can be often used as adjuvant materials, such as Indigo Naturalis (*Qingdai*) mixed with Medulla Junci (*Dengxincao*) and Cinnabaris (*Zhusha*) mixed with Poria (*Fuling*), to improve the efficacy of drugs.

4. Malaxation

This method can be used to process Caulis Bambusae in Taeniam (*Zhuru*) and Flos Eriocauli (*Gujingcao*) to facilitate prescription and preparation.

第七章　饮片切制

1. 饮片的定义

广义而言，凡是直接供中医临床调配处方或中成药生产的所有药物，统称为饮片。狭义而言，饮片是为调配处方而制成的片状药物。

2. 饮片切制的定义

将净选后的药物软化，切成一定规格的片、丝、块、段等炮制工艺，称为饮片切制。

3. 分类

切制的方法可分为手切和机器切。

4. 饮片切制的历史

饮片切制是由㕮咀发展而来，㕮咀指以口咬破。早在《五十二病方》和《内经》中就有记载。

5. 饮片切制的目的

饮片切制的目的在于：便于有效成分的煎出，利于炮炙，利于调配和制剂，便于鉴别和储存。

第一节　切制前的水处理

切制前水处理的目的是使药质地软化，易于切制，同时缓和药性，降低毒性，且去除非药用部位，清洁药物。

软化药材的原则为"少泡多润，药透水尽"。有些药材在产地趁鲜切制。还有些特殊的软化方法，如黄芩通过蒸制软化，阿胶通过烘烤软化。

1. 常用的水处理方法

常用水处理方法有淋法、淘洗法、泡法、漂法、润法。

（1）淋法

用水淋湿药材，适用于气味芳香和有效成分易随水流失的药材如薄荷、荆芥等。以药材根部软化为度。

（2）淘洗法

淘洗法是用清水洗涤或快速洗涤药物的方法。适用于质地松软、水分易渗入及有效成分易溶于水的药材，如五加皮、甘草、槟榔等。以药物洁净为度。淘洗法还要避免药材"伤水"。现多用洗药机洗涤药材。

（3）泡法

传统的泡法适用于质地坚硬。如木香、乌药等。

快速浸泡法适用于质地疏松、柔韧、易潮软的药材，如羌活；含挥发油芳香类药物或含黏液质较多的药物如当归等。以完全软化药物为度。

操作时，药物要完全浸泡在水中，浸泡的时间尽可能短些，并且视药材质地、水温、季节灵活掌握，药物大小要分档，同时要保留一定的空间以防药物吸水膨胀。

（4）漂法

本法适用于有毒性、用盐腌制过的药物及具腥臭异味的药材，如附子、川乌、海带、紫河车等。以除去其刺激性、咸味及腥臭味为度。

（5）润法

本法适用于质地较坚硬的药材。润的方法有浸润、伏润、露润。

浸润适用于质地坚硬的药材，如黄连、木香等。

伏润是将水洗的药材在密闭条件下闷润使其软化的方法。适用于质地坚硬的药物，如郁金、川芎。

露润适用于含糖、脂肪类的药材，如当归、玄参、牛膝等。还可采用蒸润、蒸汽喷雾润。

软化有两种改进的方法。真空润药法特点是可以缩短时间，并防止损害药效部位。减压冷浸法可以使水迅速进入药材组织内部，其特点是可提高药材软化的效率。

2. 药材软化程度的检查方法

弯曲法：适用于长条状药材，如白芍、山药。

指掐法：适用于团块状药物，如白术、白芷、泽泻等。

穿刺法：适用于粗大块状药物，如大黄。

手捏法：适用于不规则类药材。

剖开法：适合大块规则药材。

第二节 饮片类型及切制方法

1. 饮片类型

（1）饮片类型及规格

极薄片：厚度为0.5mm，如羚羊角。

薄片：厚度为1~2mm，如白芍。

厚片：厚度为2~4mm，如茯苓。

斜片：厚度为2~4mm，瓜子片（如桂枝），马蹄片（如大黄），柳叶片（如甘草）。

直片：厚度为2~4mm，如何首乌。

丝：细丝2~3mm，如黄柏；宽丝5~10mm，如厚朴。

段：长为10~15mm，如薄荷。

块：8~12mm³，如阿胶。

（2）切制方法

分为横切、顺切、斜切。

（3）原则

按药效部位：根、根茎类药材宜切片；角类宜切制极薄片，粉。

按质地和形状：质地致密、结实者宜切薄片，质地松泡、粉性大者宜切厚片，形体大、组织致密宜切直片，长条形宜切斜片。

2. 饮片的切制方法

分为手工切制，机器切制和其他切制。

（1）手工切制

主要有切药刀和片刀。有些用特殊的工具，如槟榔可用"蟹爪钳"切，鹿茸可用鹿茸加工壶。

（2）机器切制

主要有剁刀式切药机、旋转式切药机和多功能切药机等。

剁刀式切药机主要适用于根、根茎、全草类药材，不适用于颗粒状药材的切制。

旋转式切药机一般适用于颗粒类药物和团块类药物，不适合全草类药物。

多功能切药机主要适用于根茎、块状及果实类药材，以及多种规格斜形饮片的加工切制。

（3）其他切制

镑适用于动物角类切制，如羚羊角等。

刨适用于木质或角质坚硬类药材，如檀香、松节等。

此外，还有锉、劈、研、磨、打等方法。

第三节　饮片的干燥

1. 自然干燥

（1）特点

自然干燥的特点是不需特殊设备；适合所有饮片类型；受场地、气候限制；易污染。

（2）分类

阴干：适用于芳香类药物，如薄荷和鲜艳的颜色的药物，如红花。

晒干：适用于黏性大或糖分多地药材，如黄精；粉质类药材，如山药；油质类药材，如当归；色泽类药材，如贝母。

2. 人工干燥

（1）特点

人工干燥的特点是干燥快；不受场地、气候限制；清洁卫生；需设备、能源。

（2）设备

包括翻板式干燥机，热风式干燥机，微波干燥技术，太阳能集热干燥技术。

（3）温度

一般药物不超过80℃，含芳香挥发性成分药物一般不超过50℃为宜。

（4）湿度

干燥后的饮片含水量应控制在7%～13%。

（5）注意事项

排出干燥室中的湿气；掌握干燥时间和温度；干燥后冷却；干燥后药材含水量控制在7%～13%。

第四节　饮片的包装

1. 饮片包装的作用

（1）方便饮片的存取、运输、销售。

（2）有利于饮片的经营和防止再污染。

（3）有利于饮片的美观、清洁、卫生和定期监督检查。

（4）有利于促进饮片生产的现代化、标准化。

（5）有利于中医饮片临床调配使用。

（6）有利于中药饮片的国际贸易。

2. 饮片包装的注意事项

（1）对于贵重、毒剧药材宜用小玻璃瓶、小纸盒分装，并贴上使用说明标签。

（2）包装要注重装潢设计和 ENA 条形码。

第五节　不良因素对饮片质量的影响

1. 败片

在中药饮片切制过程中所有不符合切制规格、片形标准的饮片，都称为败片。主要包括连刀片、掉边与炸心片、皱纹片等。

（1）连刀片

是饮片之间相牵连、未完全切断的现象。系药物软化时，外部含水量过多，或刀具不锋利所致。

（2）掉边与炸心

是药材切断后，饮片内外相脱离或药材破碎的现象。系药材软化时内外软硬度不同所致。

（3）皱纹片

是饮片切面粗糙，具鱼鳞样斑痕的现象。系药材软化时水性不及，或刀具不锋利所致。

2. 翘片

饮片边缘卷曲而不平整。系药材软化时，内部含水分过多所致。

3. 变色与走味

指饮片干燥后失去原药材的色泽或失去原有的气味。系药材软化时浸泡时间太长，或干燥地方选用不当所致。

4. 走油

是药材或饮片表面有油分或黏液质渗出的现象。系药材软化时吸水量太过或环境温度多高所致。

5. 发霉

在适宜的温度和湿度条件下，因为霉菌的繁殖生长，在饮片及其炮制品表面布满菌丝的现象。

第六节　其他加工

1. 研磨

适用于矿物类药如自然铜，贝壳类药如穿山甲，果实或种子类药如栀子，小型块茎如贝母。

目的：利于有效成分的煎出；便于调配处方。

2. 制绒

麻黄可通过制成麻黄绒来减缓其作用。

3. 拌衣

青黛和朱砂可作为拌衣常用辅料，如青黛拌灯心草，朱砂拌茯苓等，可增强药效。

4. 揉搓

竹茹和谷精草可用制绒法进行炮制，便于调剂制剂。

Chapter Eight   Stir – frying

1. Definition

Stir – frying refers to the processing method that stirs and rotates the cleansed or cut drugs in a frying container constantly, if stir – frying with adjuvant materials, pre – heating the adjuvant materials before processing with the drugs.

2. Types

(1) Stir – frying without Adjuvant Materials

Stir – bake to yellow is a processing method of heating the drugs with slow or medium fire until they turn yellow or deeper in color outside, or until the drugs swell or explode to release the intrinsic odor.

Stir – bake to brown is a processing method of stir – frying the drugs with medium or strong fire until the surface of the drugs appears light brown or coke brown.

Stir – bake to charcoal is a processing method of stir – frying the drugs with strong or medium fire until the surface of the drugs appears coke brown or black.

(2) Stir – frying with Adjuvant Materials

The adjuvant materials used for processing can be bran, rice, earth, sand, clam powder, powder of talcum, etc.

3. Technics

The cleansed or cut drugs are first screened to remove ashes and separated by size. Then they are put into a pre – heated container. Adding adjuvant materials or not, the drugs are stirred or rotated constantly with different fire levels until they reach a desired degree.

4. Operating Methods

This processing can be achieved by handwork or machine. The merit of stir – frying by handwork is the simple equipment which is suitable for small – scale production. For large – scale processing, stir – frying by machine would be the better choice. The key operating points are as following: ①Stir – fry as quickly as possible during the course, and take the drugs out of the frying container in time when frying is done; ② It is suitable for processing small amounts of drugs of various kinds.

Section One　Stir – frying without Adjuvant Materials

Stir – bake to Yellow

1. Definition

Stir – bake to yellow is a processing method that stirs and rotates the cleansed or cut drugs with slow or medium fire in a frying container constantly until the surface of the drugs appears yellow or deeper in color.

2. Purposes

(1) Improve the drugs' efficacy.

(2) Reduce the drugs' toxicity and side effects.

3. Technics

Screened out ashes and separated by size, the cleansed or cut drugs are put into a preheated container. Not adding any adjuvant materials, the drugs are heated with different fire levels and stirred or rotated constantly until they reach a desired degree.

4. Standards

(1) The cutting surface turns yellowish.

(2) Color is deepened.

(3) The sound of crack could be heard.

(4) The shapes of drugs are changed or swelled.

(5) Exploding.

(6) A intrinsic odor is released.

5. Notices

When the color of the drugs turns yellowish, over – frying should be avoided. It is usually heated with slow fire while the medium fire also can be used for some special drugs, such as Fructus Xanthii (*Cangerzi*), Semen Vaccariae (*Wangbuliuxing*), Fructus Arctii (*Niubangzi*) and Semen Coicis (*Yiyiren*).

6. Suitable Drugs

Drugs made from fruits and seeds are usually processed with this method. But some drugs made from rhizomes or even animals could also be processed with this method, such as Radix Paeoniae Rubra (*Chishao*), Flos Sophorae (*Huaihua*), Aspongopus (*Jiuxiangchong*) and Os

Sepiellae seu Sepiae (*Haipiaoxiao*) .

Semen Sinapis Albae (Jiezi)

【Source】 Semen Sinapis Albae is the dried ripe seed of *Sina pis alba* L. or *Brassica juncea* (L.) Czern. et Coss. (Fam. Cruciferae) .

【Processing Methods】

1. Raw Semen Sinapis Albae　Remove impurities and pound drugs into powders.

2. Stir－frying Semen Sinapis Albae　Put the cleansed drugs into a frying container, heat with mild fire and stir－fry them until the drugs' color deepens, the sound of crack is heard, and the drugs become yellowish on the cutting surface and emit a fragrant odor.

【Processing Functions】

1. Raw Semen Sinapis Albae　The raw drug is strong in dispersing and good at activating meridians to relieve pain. It can be used in treating symptoms of oppression in chest, painful ribs, joints, sores and ulcers.

2. Stir－fried Semen Sinapis Albae　The processing can moderate the drug's nature of dispersing to avoid consuming the *qi* and damaging the *yin*. And it also can warm the lung to eliminate phlegm so it is usually used to treat phlegm and cough. For example, it can be used in Sanzi Yangqin Decoction (recorded in *Han's Clear View of Medicine*) .

【Processing Purposes】

1. Moderate the nature of dispersing and avoid consuming the *qi* and damaging the *yin*.

2. Facilitate the crushing and decoction.

3. Inactivate the enzymes and protect the glycosides.

4. Keep the effective components from being damaged.

5. Be suitable for various clinical application.

【Processing Research】

There are thioglycoside compounds in the drugs, especially mustard glycoside, which can be enzymolysis to release mustard oil with the effects of assisting digestion and removing phlegm. After being stir－fried, the myrosinase would be destroyed and the mustard glycoside could remain. Mustard glycoside decomposes slowly in the stomach and intestines and releases mustard oil gradually to achieve the function of stopping cough and removing phlegm.

Semen Ziziphi Spinosae (Suanzaoren)

【Source】 Semen Ziziphi Spinosae is the dried ripe seed of *Ziziphus jujuba Mill. var. spinosa* (Bunge) Hu ex H. F. Chou (Fam. Rhamnaceae) .

【Processing Methods】

1. Raw Semen Ziziphi Spinosae　Remove impurities and pound drugs into powders.

2. Stir－frying Semen Ziziphi Spinosae　Put the cleansed drugs into a frying container, heat with slow fire and stir－fry them quickly until the drugs swell, deepen in color, crack, become yellowish on the cutting surface and emit a fragrant odor.

【Processing Functions】

1. Raw Semen Ziziphi Spinosae

The raw drug has the functions of nourishing the heart and calming the mind. So it is often used in treating syndromes of palpitations due to fright, poor memory, vertigo and insomnia caused by deficiency of heart *yin* and liver – kidney depletion. For example, it can be used in Suanzaoren Decoction (recorded in *Synopsis Golden Chamber*).

2. Stir – fried Semen Ziziphi Spinosae

The effect of nourishing the heart and calming the mind of stir – fried drug is better than that of raw drug. It can be used in formulas such as Support Heart Decoction (recorded in *Fine Formulas*) to treat symptoms of palpitations, poor memory, insomnia and profuse dreaming caused by heart and blood deficiency.

【Processing Purposes】

1. The testa of the Raw Spine Date Seed will dehisce after being fried, making it easier to be crushed and decocted. The content of effective components is 17. 4% in fried drugs, 16. 2% in raw drugs, and 13. 8% in charred drugs.

2. The effect of tranquilization is strengthened after being processed.

【Processing Research】

It is reported that the raw and stir – fried Spine Date Seed have the same effect of nourishing the heart and calming the mind while the charred drugs would lose this effect.

Semen Pharbitidis (Qianniuzi)

【Source】 Semen Pharbitidis is the dried ripe seed of *Pharbitis nil* (L.) Choisy or *Pharbitis pupurea* (L.) Voigt (Fam. Convolvulaceae).

【Processing Methods】

1. Raw Semen Pharbitidis

Remove impurities and pound the drug into powders.

2. Stir – frying Semen Pharbitidis

Put the cleansed drugs into a frying container, heat with mild fire and stir – fry them until the drugs swell, deepen in color, crack, become yellowish on the cutting surface and emit a fragrant odor.

【Processing Functions】

1. Raw Semen Pharbitidis

The raw drug has the functions of purging urine and removing stagnation, eliminating phlegm and removing rheum, and killing worms. For example, it can be used in Zhouche Pills to treat polyhydramnios (recorded in *The Complete Works of Zhang Jing – yue*).

2. Stir – fried Semen Pharbitidis

Stir – fried drug is often used in treating food accumulation syndrome, *qi* counter flow and phlegm coagulation. For example, it can be used in Yinianjin in treating children's bad appetite, stagnation, constipation and phlegm panting (recorded in *Chinese Pharmacopoeia*).

【Processing Purposes】

1. Reduce toxicity and moderate the nature of the drug.

2. Make the drug crisper in texture and help the extraction of the effective components.

3. Be suitable for various clinical application.

【Processing Research】

There are pharbitisin and alkaloids in Pharbitidis seed. The pharbitisin has the function of irritating the intestinal tract, which can increase enterokinesia. After being stir – fried, the content of pharbitisin will be reduced and the functions of promoting urine and defecation would be moderated.

Fructus Xanthii （Cangerzi）

【Source】 Fructus Xanthii is the dried ripe bur with involucre of *Xanthium sibiricum* Patr. （Fam. Compositae）.

【Processing Methods】

1. Raw Fructus Xanthii Remove impurities and pound the drug into powders.

2. Stir – frying Fructus Xanthii Put the cleansed drugs into a frying container, heat with medium fire and stir – fry them until the drug's outer part becomes yellowish and the spine is scorched. Then remove the spine and screen out the impurities.

【Processing Functions】

1. Raw Fructus Xanthii The raw drug has the functions of removing wind – damp and relieving itching.

2. Stir – fried Fructus Xanthii The processing can reduce the toxicity and make the drug good at relieving stuffy nose, expelling wind – damp and relieving pain.

【Processing Purposes】

1. Reduce the toxicity.

2. Make it easy to remove the spine.

【Processing Research】

The toxic component in the Raw Siberian Cocklebur Fruit would be denatured after being stir – fried so that the toxicity would be reduced. At the same time, because of the medium heat during stir – frying, the spine would be removed easily and the relative content of effective components will be increased, thus the drug's effectiveness would be increased.

Semen Raphani （Laifuzi）

【Source】 Semen Raphani is the dried ripe seed of *Raphanus sativus* L. （Fam. Cruciferae）.

【Processing Methods】

1. Raw Semen Raphani Remove impurities and pound the drug into powders.

2. Stir – frying Semen Raphani Put the cleansed drugs into a frying container, heat with mild fire and stir – fry them until the drugs swell and the sound of cracking becomes weaker. Take them out when the drugs become easy to be crushed by hands, yellowish on the cutting surface, and have a fragrant odor.

【Processing Functions】

1. Raw Semen Raphani The raw drug has the nature of ascending and scattering; good at causing wind – phlegm vomiting.

2. Stir – fried Semen Raphani The processing can transform the drug's nature of ascending to descending, which makes it good at removing food stagnation, relieving distension directing *qi* downward and dissolving phlegm. For example, it can be used in Sanzi Yangqin Decoction to treat panting and cough (recorded in *Formulas to Protect the Original Qi*), and in Harmony – Preserving Pill to treat food stagnation (recorded in *Chinese Pharmacopoeia*).

【Processing Purposes】

1. Moderate the nature of the drug and eliminate toxicity and side effects.

2. Make it easy to be crushed and decocted to enhance the effectiveness.

Semen Coicis (Yiyiren)

【Source】 Semen Coicis is the dried ripe kernel of *Coix lacryma – jobi* L. var. *mayuen* (Roman.) Stapf (Fam. Gramineae).

【Processing Methods】

1. Raw Semen Coicis Remove impurities and screen out ashes of the drug.

2. Stir – frying Semen Coicis Put the drugs in a frying container, heat with medium fire and stir – fry them until the drugs become yellowish, swell slightly and have a little enation on the surface.

3. Stir – frying Semen Coicis with Bran Put the bran into a preheated frying pan, which will produce smokes immediately. Then put the raw drugs into the pan and stir – fry them together quickly until the drugs become yellowish and swell. Take them out and screen out the bran. In this procedure, use 15kg bran for 100kg drugs.

【Processing Functions】

1. Raw Semen Coicis The raw drug is cold in nature and good at inducing diuresis and draining damp, clearing heat to eliminate pus and removing arthralgia to relieve pain.

2. Processed Semen Coicis The processing can moderate the drug's nature of coldness, which makes it good at fortifying the spleen and arresting diarrhea. So it can be used in treating diarrhea due to spleen deficiency, bad appetite and food stagnation. For example, it is used in Shenling Baizhu Powder (recorded in *Chinese Pharmacopoeia*).

Semen Vaccariae (Wangbuliuxing)

【Source】 Semen Vaccariae is the dried ripe seed of *Vaccaria segetalis* (Neck.) Garcke (Fam. Caryophyllaceae).

【Processing Methods】

1. Raw Semen Vaccariae Remove impurities, cleanse it before drying.

2. Stir – frying Semen Vaccariae Put the cleansed drugs into a preheated pan with medium fire and stir – fry them quickly until most of the drugs explode.

【Processing Functions】

1. Raw Semen Vaccariae The raw drug is good at subduing inflammation. So it can be used in Cowherb Seed Powder (recorded in *Yixinfang*) to treat inflammations such as acute mastitis.

2. Stir – fried Semen Vaccariae   Stir – frying makes the drug's texture soft and loose so as to help the extraction of the effective components. The stir – fried drug is good at activating blood to promote menstruation; promoting lactation and relieving strangury. For example, it can be used in Tongru Siwu Decoction (recorded in *Six Texts on Medical Essentials – Yilüeliushu*) .

【Processing Purposes】

1. Facilitate extracting the effective component.

2. Enlarge the applying scope.

【Processing Research】

The drug's effect has close relationship with the extraction of effective components while the content of extraction is determined by the process of frying and explosion. At different stages of processing such as raw drugs, fried drugs without explosion, fried drugs with a little explosion and fried drugs with complete explosion, the extraction in water would be 7. 11% , 8. 58% , 11. 56% and 14. 39% respectively; When the rates of explosion are 60% , 70% , 80% , 90% and 100% , the content of extraction would be 11. 69% , 12. 36% , 13. 11% , 13. 80% and 14. 39% respectively. The higher the explosion rate, the higher the extraction rate.

Parching

1. Definition

It is a processing method of stir – frying the cleansed or cut drugs with medium or strong fire until they are parched.

2. Purposes

(1) Strengthen the drugs' effects of fortifying the spleen and promoting digestion. Fructus Hordei Germinatus (*Maiya*), Fructus Setariae Germinatus (*Guya*) and Massa Medicata Fermentata (*Shenqu*) are good examples.

(2) Moderate the nature of drugs and reduce the irritating nature of drugs. Such as Semen Arecae (*Binglang*) Fructus Gardeniae (*Zhizi*) and Fructus Meliae Toosendan (*Chuanlianzi*) .

3. Technics

Screened out ashes and separated by size, the cleansed or cut drugs are put into a preheated container. Not adding any adjuvant materials, the drugs are heated with different fire levels and stirred or rotated constantly until they reach a desired degree.

4. Standards

(1) For the drugs such as Fructus Crataegi (*Shanzha*) and Massa Medicata Fermentata (*Shenqu*), the color turns coke brown outside and coke yellow inside.

(2) For the drugs such as Fructus Crataegi (*Shanzha*) and Fructus Setariae Germinatus (*Guya*), the color turns coke yellow outside and a deeper color inside.

5. Notice

When stir – frying the drugs to be parched, avoid being charred.

6. Suitable Drugs

Drugs that have the functions of fortifying the spleen to promote digestion can be processed with this method. And drugs that cause irritation to intestines and stomach also can be stir – fried to be parched.

Fructus Gardeniae (Zhizi)

【Source】 Fructus Gardeniae is the dried ripe fruit of *Gardenia jasminoides* Ellis (Fam. Rubiaceae).

【Processing Methods】

1. Raw Fructus Gardeniae Remove impurities and grind the drug.

2. Stir – frying Fructus Gardeniae Put the fragmented drugs into a frying pan and heat with slow fire until the drugs' outer part turns dark yellow.

3. Parching Fructus Gardeniae Put the fragmented drugs into a frying pan and heat with medium fire until the drugs' outer part turns coke yellow.

4. Charring Fructus Gardeniae Put the fragmented drugs into a frying pan and heat with strong fire until the drugs' outer part becomes pitchy. Then spray a little water to extinguish sparkles.

【Processing Functions】

1. Raw Fructus Gardeniae The raw drug is bitter and cold in nature and good at draining fire and dampness, cooling blood and resolving toxins. For example, it can be used in Coptidis Decoction for detoxification to treat warm disease, high heat, vexation and agitation, unconsciousness, and delirious speech (recorded in *The Collections on Treating Deficieny – Consumption*) or in Yinchenhao Decoction to treat jaundice caused by damp – heat (recorded in *Treatise on Cold Damage and Miscellaneous Diseases*). It also can be grinded to mix with wheat powder and yellow wine to treat bruises, sprains, and swellings.

2. Parched Fructus Gardeniae The drug's bitter and cold nature are moderated, and it can be used to clear away heat and dysphoria.

3. Charred Fructus Gardeniae The charred drug is a little bitter and cold in nature. It is good at cooling blood to stop bleeding. For example, it can be used in Shihui Powder (recorded in *Ten Medicinal Formulas*).

【Processing Purposes】

1. Bring new functions and enhance the drug's original efficacy.

2. Moderate the nature of the drugs.

【Processing Research】

There are other processing methods for Cape Jasmine Fruit, such as being stir – fried with ginger juice or decorticated. Whatever the processing method is, the content of geniposide and ur-solic acid would be decreased and thus the pharmacological action would be affected and changed. For example, the effects of cholagogue, hemostasis, abatement of fever and bacteriostasis would be different after being processed with different methods. For example, Parched Cape Jasmine Fruit has the strongest effects on sedation and hemostasis.

Fructus Crataegi (Shanzha)

【Source】 Fructus Crataegi is the dried ripe fruit of *Crataegus pinnatifida* Bge. var *major* N. E. Br. , or *Crataegus pinnatifida* Bge. (Fam. Rosaceae) .

【Processing Methods】

1. Raw Fructus Crataegi   Remove impurities, fallen nucleus and carpopodium of the drug.

2. Stir – frying Fructus Crataegi   Put the cleansed drugs in a frying container, heat with medium fire and stir – fry them until the color of the drugs turns deeper.

3. Parching Fructus Crataegi   Put the cleansed drugs in a frying container, heat with medium fire and stir – fry them until the drugs turn coke brown outside and coke yellow inside.

4. Carbonizing Fructus Crataegi   Put the cleansed drugs in a frying container, heat with strong fire and stir – fry them until the drugs turn coke black outside and coke brown inside.

【Processing Functions】

1. Raw Fructus Crataegi   The raw drug can activate blood and resolve stasis.

2. Stir – fried Fructus Crataegi   Frying can moderate the drug's sour taste and irritation to the stomach, which enhances the effect of promoting digestion and removing stagnation. Stir – fried drugs can be used for splenic asthenia, dyspeptic retention, poor appetite, low spirit and lack of strength.

3. Parched Fructus Crataegi   This method can moderate the drug's sour taste and increase the bitterness, which makes it good at promoting digestion and arresting diarrhea. So parched drugs are often used to treat food stagnation, the spleen deficiency and diarrhea. For example, it can be used in Baohe Pills to treat food stagnation (recorded in *Chinese Pharmacopoeia*) .

4. Carbonized Fructus Crataegi   Charred drug is astringent in taste and has the functions of stanching bleeding and arresting diarrhea.

【Processing Research】

The content of organic acid is the highest in the raw drugs, less in stir – fried drugs and the least in parched drugs. That is to say, the content of the organic acid would be decreased by 68% through processing. Besides, the raw drugs and stir – fried drugs have stronger effect in promoting digestion than other processed drugs. And the antibiosis of the raw drugs and parched drugs is stronger than the other processed drugs.

Semen Arecae (Binglang)

【Source】 Semen Arecae is the dried ripe seed of *Areca catechu* L. (Fam. Palmae) .

【Processing Methods】

1. Raw Semen Arecae Clean and immerse the seeds in water to become soft, cut the seeds into thin slices, air drying.

2. Stir – frying Semen Arecae Put the sliced drugs in a frying container, heat with mild fire and stir – fry them until the outer part turns yellowish.

3. Parching Semen Arecae Put the sliced drugs in a frying container, heat with medium fire and stir – fry them until the outer part turns coke yellow.

4. Carbonizing Semen Arecae Put the sliced drugs in a frying container, heat with strong fire and stir – fry them until the outer part turns burned black.

【Processing Functions】

1. Raw Semen Arecae The raw drug has the functions of killing parasites, dispersing food accumulation, directing *qi* downward, promoting urination and preventing attack of malaria.

2. Stir – fried Semen Arecae Frying can moderate the nature of drugs, reduce side – effects, promote digestion, and remove food stagnation.

3. Parched Semen Arecae This processing can moderate the nature of drugs, strengthen the effects of promoting digestion and removing food stagnation. It can be used in Kaixiong Shunqi Pills (recorded in *Handbook of Proprietary Chinese Medicine Preparations*).

4. Carbonized Semen Arecae Charred drug is good at stanching bleeding.

【Processing Purposes】

1. Strengthen drug efficacy and moderate the nature of drugs.

2. Be suitable for more clinical application.

【Processing Research】

When processing the raw drug, the principle of 'less soaking, more moistening' should be adopted to avoid the loss of effective components. The research shows that the content of arecaline in raw drugs and stir – fried drugs are 0. 4% ~ 0. 52% and 0. 13% ~ 0. 31% respectively. And the loss of the alkaloid is 24% after being soaked, reducing the effect of insecticide. Meanwhile, the drugs should be dried in open air rather than under the sun and the heat level should be lower than usual when charring.

Carbonizing by stir – frying

1. Definition

It is a method of stir – frying the drugs to a carbonized state with strong or medium fire.

2. Purposes

(1) Strengthen or bring the drugs' effect of hemostasis. Radix Sanguisorbae (*Diyu*) and Pollen Typhae (*Puhuang*) are good examples.

(2) Strengthen the drugs' effect of arresting diarrhea. Dark Plum Fruit (*Wumei*) and Pericarpium Granati (*Shiliupi*) are good examples.

3. Technics

Screened out ashes and separated by size, the cleansed or cut drugs are put into a preheated container. Not adding any adjuvant materials, the drugs are heated with different fire levels and stirred or rotated constantly until they reach a desired degree. Then spray some water to extinguish sparkles.

4. Standards

（1）For the drugs made from roots and tubers, stir – fry them until the drugs turn coke black or coke brown outside.

（2）For the drugs made from flowers or leaves and herbs, stir – fry them until "burned as charcoal while function preserved".

（3）For the drugs such as Indian Radix Rubiae（*Qiancao*）, stir – fry them until the drugs turn black and burnished.

5. Notices

（1）Different fire levels should be applied according to different drugs. For example, strong fire should be used to heat drugs with hard texture, while medium fire can be applied to heat drugs with soft texture such as drugs made from flower, pollen, leaf or grass.

（2）Spray water to extinguish sparkles to avoid the drugs being burnt thoroughly.

（3）Functions of drugs should be preserved when they are carbonized by stir – frying.

（4）Store after being cooled to avoid recrudescence.

6. Suitable Drugs

The method can be used to process drugs with effects of hemostasis and arresting diarrhea.

Radix Sanguisorbae（Diyu）

【Source】 Radix Sanguisorbae is the dried root of *Sanguisorba officinalis* L. or *Sanguisorba officinalis* L. var. *longifolia*（Bert. ）Yü et Li（Fam. Rosaceae）.

【Processing Methods】

1. Raw Radix Sanguisorbae   Clear away the twigs and cut it into chunks.

2. Carbonizing Radix Sanguisorbae   Put the sliced drugs into a preheated frying pan, heat with strong fire and stir – fry them quickly until the drugs turn burned black outside and sepia inside.

【Processing Functions】

1. Raw Radix Sanguisorbae   The raw drug can cool blood, resolve toxins, and relieve pain.

2. Carbonized Radix Sanguisorbae   Carbonized drug can astringe and stanch bleeding. For example, it can be used in treating scalds and burns.

【Processing Purposes】

1. Strengthen the effect of hemostasis.

2. Be suitable for more clinical application.

【Processing Research】

After being carbonized by stir – frying, the drugs have the pharmacologic action of hemostasis and bacteriostasis, and can be used in treating burns and scalds.

Rhizoma Zingiberis (Ganjiang)

【Source】 Rhizoma Zingiber is the dried rhizome of *Zingiber of ficinale* (Willd.) Rosc. (Fam. Zingiberaceae) .

【Processing Methods】

1. Raw Rhizoma Zingiberis   Remove impurities and cut the drug into thick pieces or sections.

2. Frying Rhizoma Zingiberis   Put the clean river sand into a frying container first. Then heat with strong fire, put pieces or sections of the drugs into the container and stir – fry them together constantly until the drug's outer part swells and the color turns sepia.

3. Carbonizing Rhizoma Zingiberis   Put sections of drugs into a frying container, heat with strong fire and stir – fry them quickly until the drugs turn burned black outside and sepia inside. Then, spray water to extinguish sparkle.

Notice: Ventilate when processing, fry until smoking stops and cool quickly.

【Processing Functions】

1. Raw Rhizoma Zingiberis   The raw drug is pungent in taste and hot in nature. And it has the functions of warming the interior for dispelling cold, restoring *yang* from collapse, and drying dampness and dispersing phlegm.

2. Stir – fried Rhizoma Zingiberis   The stir – fried drug is weaker in the nature of pungent compared with the raw drug, and good at warming meridians to stop bleeding.

3. Carbonized Rhizoma Zingiberis   The carbonized drug is bitter, astringent in taste, and warm in nature. It has the functions of warming the center and dispelling cold, warming the meridian and stanching bleeding. It can be used in Aconite Center – Regulating Pill and Sages Powder to treat metrorrhagia (recorded in *Teachings of Zhu Danxi*) .

【Processing Purpose】

1. Facilitate the extraction of the effective components.

2. Be suitable for more clinical application.

【Processing Research】

In these three types of Zingiberis, the content of volatile oil is the highest in raw drugs, less in fried drugs and the least in carbonized drugs. And the processed drugs can do better in treating ulcers and stopping bleeding.

Pollen Typhae (Puhuang)

【Source】 Pollen Typhae is the dried pollen of *Typha angustifolia* L. , *Typha orientalis* Presl or other plants of the same genus (Fam. Typhaceae) .

【Processing Methods】

1. Raw Pollen Typhae Rub dry pollen to powder and remove filament and impurities.

2. Carbonizing Pollen Typhae Put the cleansed drugs in a frying container, heat with medium fire and stir – fry them until the drug turns sepia. Then spray water to extinguish sparkles.

Notices: The fire should be controled to avoid burning the drugs to ashes. And the drugs should be cooled thoroughly before storage.

【Processing Functions】

1. Raw Pollen Typhae The raw drug is sweet in taste and plain in nature and has the functions of promoting blood circulation, removing blood stasis and relieving pain. It can be used in Lower Abdominal Stasis – Expelling Decoction.

2. Carbonized Pollen Typhae The Carbonized drug is astringent in nature and can enhance the effect of hemostasis. It can be used in Sihong Pills.

【Processing Purposes】

Raw drugs can promote blood circulation while carbonized drugs are good at stanching bleeding. So the processing can not only change the nature of the drugs but also change clinical uses.

【Processing Research】

Compared with raw drugs, the carbonized drugs have a stronger effect on restraining fibrinolysin. According to the pharmacological tests, the carbonized drugs can increase blood coagulation in mice, meaning that carbonizing can guarantee the drugs' effect of hemostasis.

Section Two　Stir – frying with Adjuvant Materials

Stir – frying with Wheat Bran

1. Definition

It is a method of stir – frying the cleansed or cut drugs with wheat bran, usually with medium fire.

2. Purposes

(1) Reduce the content of volatile oil.

(2) Heat the drugs.

(3) Provide sufficient time or heat in processing.

(4) Remove the bad odor and modify the drugs' taste.

(5) Strengthen the drug's effects of tonifying *qi* and harmonizing the center, astringing the intestines and checking diarrhea.

3. Technics

Preheat a pan with medium or strong fire and sprinkle the bran into it evenly. Add the drugs in when the bran smokes and stir – fry them together quickly until the drugs become yellow and the bran turns black.

4. Amount of Adjuvant Material

Use 10 ~ 15kg wheat bran for 100kg drugs.

5. Suitable Drugs

This method can be used to process drugs with the effect of tonifying the spleen and stomach, or drugs with strong effects and fishy odor.

6. Notices

(1) Preheat the pan with medium fire.
(2) Sprinkle the bran evenly.
(3) Dry the drugs before processing.
(4) Take the drugs out quickly when they are stir – fried to a desired degree.

Fructus Aurantii (Zhiqiao)

【Source】Fructus Aurantii is the dried, immature fruit of *Citrus auranitium* L. and its cultivated varieties (Fam. Rutaceae).

【Processing Methods】

1. Raw Fructus Aurantii Remove impurities, clean and moisten the raw drug thoroughly, discard kernel, and cut it into thin slices. It is creamy – white and has a nice odor.

2. Stir – frying Fructus Aurantii with Bran First, preheat a pan and sprinkle a certain amount of the bran into the pan evenly. Then heat with medium fire, add drugs in when the bran smokes and stir – fry them constantly until the drugs turn pale yellow and the bran becomes black. Use 10kg bran per 100kg drugs.

【Processing Functions】

1. Raw Fructus Aurantii The raw drug is pungent in nature and good at relieving stagnation of *qi*. For example, it can be used in Xuefu Zhuyu Decoction.

2. Stir – fried Fructus Aurantii Processing with bran can moderate the pungent nature of the drug, which makes it good at rectifying *qi*, fortifying, and promoting digestion. For example, it can be used in Muxiang Binglang Pills to treat food stagnation and fullness of stomach cavity.

【Processing Purposes】

1. Moderate the drug's nature.

2. Enlarge clinical usage.

【Processing Research】

The content of volatile oil in the drug is reduced after they are processed with bran so that the irritating character is moderated and the effect of invigorating the stomach is strengthened. Because most of the volatile oil and effective components exist in the peel, the flesh containing little useful components should be discarded.

Rhizoma Atractylodis (Cangzhu)

【Source】 Rhizoma Atractylodis is the dried rhizome of *Atractylodes lancea* (Thunb.) DC. or *Atractylodes chinensis* (DC.) Koidz. (Fam. Compositae).

【Processing Methods】

1. Raw Rhizoma Atractylodis　Remove impurities, soak the raw drug in water, clean and moisten it thoroughly, and cut it into thick slices.

2. Stir – frying Rhizoma Atractylodis with Bran　Preheat a pan, put the bran into it evenly and heat with medium fire. Add drugs in when the bran smokes and stir – fry them together quickly until the drugs turn deep yellow. Use 10kg bran per 100kg drugs.

3. Parching Rhizoma Atractylodis　Preheat the pan, stir – fry the sliced drugs with medium fire until the drugs turn coke brown.

【Processing Functions】

1. Raw Rhizoma Atractylodis　The raw drugs can eliminate wind and diaphoresis and remove coldness. It can be used for treating wind – dampness and painful bi. For example, it can be used in the decoction of Coicis Semen (*Yiyiren*) to treat wind – dampness and arthralgia.

2. Stir – frying Rhizoma Atractylodis with Bran　The nature of pungent and dryness of this product is moderated while the fragrant odor is increased. The processing strengthens the effect of fortifying the spleen and harmonizing the stomach.

3. Parched Rhizoma Atractylodis　The processing can moderate the drug's nature of pungent and dryness greatly, which makes it have the main effect of astringing the intestines and arresting. For example, it can be used in Jiaozhu Pills (recorded in *The Collections for Saving Lives*).

【Processing Research】

The main components in volatile oil are atractylol and atractylone. After stir – frying drugs with the bran, the content of atractylol and atractylone are reduced greatly, and the nature of pungent and dryness is moderated.

Bombyx Batryticatus (Jiangcan)

【Source】 Bombyx Batryticatus is the dried body of the 4 ~ 5th stage larva of *Bombyx mori* Linnaeus. (Fam. Bombycidae) died of infection (or artificial infection) of *Beauveria bassiana* (Bals.) Vuill ant.

【Processing Methods】

1. Raw Bombyx Batryticatus　Remove impurities and silk, then clean and dry the drug under the sun.

2. Stir – frying Bombyx Batryticatus with Bran   Heat a pan with medium fire and put a certain amount of bran into it evenly. Add drugs in when the bran smokes and stir – fry them together quickly until the drugs turn yellow outside. Use 10kg bran per 100kg drugs.

【Processing Functions】

1. Raw Bombyx Batryticatus   The raw drug is good at dispelling wind and fright, dissolving phlegm and dissipating masses. It can be used for headache due to pathogenic wind heat.

2. Stir – frying Bombyx Batryticatus with Bran   The processing makes the drug good at dissolving phlegm and dissipating masses. It can be used in treating loss of voice caused by stroke. For example, it is used in Silkworm Larva Powder to treat swollen and sore throat.

【Processing Purposes】

1. Clean the drugs.

2. Keep or strengthen the efficacy.

3. Remove the bad odor and taste to facilitate taking.

4. Destroy the microbes on the surface.

Stir – frying with Rice

1. Definition

It is a method of stir – frying the cleaned and cut drugs with rice to a certain degree, usually with medium fire.

2. Functions

(1) Indicate the degrees of processing.

(2) Heat drugs.

(3) Absorb the toxic components.

(4) Strengthen the effect of fortifying the spleen and arresting diarrhea.

3. Technics

Put the rice into a preheated pan first and heat with medium fire until the rice smokes. Then add drugs into the pan and stir quickly until the drugs' color turns deeper or the rice's color becomes coke yellow or coke brown.

4. Amount of Adjuvant Material

Use 20kg rice for 100kg drugs.

5. Suitable Drugs

This method can be used to process toxic drugs (Mylabris – *Banmao*) and drugs with the effect of tonifying the spleen and boosting *qi* (Radix Codonopsis – *Dangshen*) .

6. Notices

（1）When processing insect drugs, pay attention to the color change of the rice.

（2）When processing plant drugs, pay attention to the color change of the drug.

Radix Codonopsis（Dangshen）

【Source】Radix Codonopsis is the dried root of *Codonopsis pilosula*（Franch. ）Nannf. , *Codonopsis pilosula* Nannf. var. *modesta*（Nannf. ）L. T. Shen or *Codonopsis tangshen* Oliv.（Fam. Campanulaceae）.

【Processing Methods】

1. Raw Radix Codonopsis
Remove impurities, clean and moisten the drugs, and cut them into thick pieces.

2. Stir – frying Radix Codonopsis with Rice
Put the rice into a preheated frying pan and heat with medium fire until the rice smokes. Add the drugs in and stir – fry them together until the drugs become yellow. Use 20kg rice per 100kg drugs.

3. Stir – frying Radix Codonopsis with Honey
First, dilute the refined honey with water and mix it with the pieces of *Dangshen* thoroughly. Then put them into a preheat pan with mild fire and stir – fry them quickly until the drugs turn yellowish – brown outside and not sticking. Use 20kg honey per 100kg *Dangshen*.

【Processing Functions】

1. Raw Radix Codonopsis
The raw drug is good at boosting *qi* and engendering fluid. For example, it can be used in Decoction of Nourishing Lung which is suitable for deficiency of both *qi* and *yin*. Another prescription is Liangyi Ointment which is suitable for deficiency of both *qi* and blood（recorded in *The Collections of the Formulas*）.

2. Stir – frying Radix Codonopsis with Rice
The processing makes the drug have a nicer odor, and can strengthen the effects of regulating the stomach, fortifying the spleen and arresting diarrhea. For example, it can be used in Shenqi Baizhu Decoction, which has the effect of supplementing the center and replenishing *qi*, or in Lizhong Decoction which can treat diarrhea caused by deficiency of spleen.

3. Stir – frying Radix Codonopsis with Honey
Processing with honey can strengthen the effects of supplementing the center, boosting *qi*, nourishing *yin* and relieving dryness.

【Processing Research】

According to some researches, the content of effective components is higher in thick pieces than in other shapes.

Mylabris（Banmao）

【Source】Mylabris is the dried body of *Mylabris phalerata* Pallas or *Mylabris cichorii* Linnaeus（Fam. Meloidae）.

【Processing Methods】

1. Raw Mylabris   Discard the drugs' head, feet, wings and impurities.

2. Stir – frying Mylabris with Rice   Put the rice into a preheated pan and heat with medium fire until the rice smokes. Add drugs in and stir – fry them together quickly until the rice turns brown. Use 20kg rice per 100kg drugs.

【Processing Functions】

1. Raw Mylabris   The raw drug is good at counteracting toxic substances and phagedena. It can be used in treating obstinate dermatomycosis.

2. Stir – frying Mylabris with Rice   The stir – fried drug can remove obstruction in meridians, destroy the excess foods and eliminates stagnation. For example, it can be used in Banmao Tongjing Pills to treat extravasated blood and menstrual occlusion (recorded in *A Compendium of Female Disorders*).

【Processing Purposes】

1. Reduce toxicity and improve the effectiveness.

2. Rice is an index of the processing degree.

【Processing Research】

The main toxic component in Blister Beetle is cantharides camphor which starts to sublimate at 84℃ and reaches the sublimation point at 110℃. The temperature of the frying pan when processing with rice should be 128℃, which is suitable for the sublimation of cantharides camphor. After being stir – fried with rice, the drugs' toxicity would be reduced as the contents of toxic cantharides camphor are decreased.

When heating, too high temperature should be avoided so as not to cause charring. Ventilation and poison prevention are also necessary. Hands should be washed immediately after processing.

Stir – frying with Soil

1. Definition

It is a method of stir – frying the cleaned or cut drugs with soil to a certain degree, normally with medium fire.

2. Function

Processing with soil can strengthen the effects of tonifying the spleen and arresting diarrhea.

3. Technics

Grind the soil and put it into a pan, heating with medium fire. Stir – fry the soil to be loose and smooth. Add the drugs in and stir – fry them together until the drugs' surface is evenly covered with soil. When there is an aroma, take them out and screen out the soil.

4. Amount of Adjuvant Material

25 ~ 30kg soil for 100kg drugs.

5. Suitable Drugs

This method can be used to process drugs with the effects of tonifying the spleen and arresting diarrhea.

Rhizoma Atractylodis Macrocephalae（Baizhu）

【Source】 Rhizoma Atractylod is Macrocephalae is the dried rhizome of *Atractylodes macrocephala* Koidz.（Fam. Compositae）.

【Processing Methods】

1. Raw Rhizoma Atractylodis Macrocephalae　Remove impurities, clean and moisten them thoroughly in water, and cut them into thick pieces.

2. Stir – frying Rhizoma Atractylodis Macrocephalae with Soil　Put the soil into a pan and heat it to be loose and smooth with medium fire. Add the drugs in and stir – fry them together. Take them out when the drugs are covered with soil evenly. Use 25kg soil for 100kg drugs.

3. Stir – frying Rhizoma Atractylodis Macrocephalae with Bran　Put the bran into a preheated pan with medium fire and add drugs in when the bran smokes. Then stir – fry them together constantly until the drugs' outer part turns yellow with a coke aroma. Use 10kg bran for 100kg drugs.

【Processing Functions】

1. Raw Rhizoma Atractylodis Macrocephalae　The raw drug can fortify the spleen, remove dampness and induce diuresis and detumescence.

2. Stir – frying Rhizoma Atractylodis Macrocephalae with Soil　The drug processed with this method is good at replenishing the spleen and arresting diarrhea.

3. Stir – frying Rhizoma Atractylodis Macrocephalae with Bran　Stir – frying with the bran can moderate the drug's nature of dryness, fortify the spleen and regulate the stomach.

【Processing Purposes】

1. Moderate drugs' dryness.

2. Enlarge the clinical applications.

3. Enhance drugs' effectiveness.

【Processing Research】

After being stir – fried with the soil, the content of volatile oil is reduced and the dryness is moderated.

Rhizoma Dioscoreae（Shanyao）

【Source 】 Rhizoma Dioscoreae is the dried rhizome of *Dioscorea opposite* Thunb.（Fam. Dioscoreaceae）.

【Processing Methods】

1. Raw Rhizoma Dioscoreae　· Remove impurities, separate them by size, clean and moisten them, and cut them into thick pieces.

2. Stir – frying Rhizoma Dioscoreae with Soil   Put the soil into a pan and heat it to be loose and smooth with medium fire. Add the drugs in and stir – fry them with the soil. Take them out when the drugs are covered with soil evenly. Use 30kg soil for 100kg drugs.

3. Stir – frying Rhizoma Dioscoreae with Bran   Put the bran into a heated pan and add the drugs in when the bran smokes. Stir – fry them constantly with medium fire until the drugs' outer part turns yellow with a coke aroma. Use 10kg bran per 100kg drugs.

【Processing Functions】

1. Raw Rhizoma Dioscoreae   The raw drug mainly has the functions of tonifying kidney to produce essence and benefiting lung *yin*. For example, it can be used in Six – Drug Rehmannia Pill.

2. Stir – frying Rhizoma Dioscoreae with Soil   Stir – frying with the soil can make the drug has the functions of tonifying the spleen and arresting diarrhea.

3. Stir – frying Rhizoma Dioscoreae with Bran   Stir – frying with the bran can make the drug has the functions of supplementing the spleen and invigorating the stomach.

【Processing Research】

In raw drugs, drugs stir – fried without adjuvant materials, drugs stir – fried with soil and those stir – fried with bran, the contents of diosgenin are 11.69%, 12.36%, 13.11% and 13.80% respectively. This result indicates that after being stir – fried, the content of effective components would be increased and thus the effect would be enhanced.

The suitable seasons to process this drugs should be spring or autumn. Dry drugs in time to avoid rotting. The soil should be renewed frequently to ensure the effectiveness of the drugs.

Stir – frying with Sand

1. Definition

It is a method of stir – frying the cleaned or cut drugs with hot sand to a certain degree, usually heating with strong fire.

2. Functions

(1) Help compounding and preparing.

(2) Facilitate removing the hair of the drug.

(3) Reduce toxicity.

(4) Modify the bad taste and odor.

3. Technics

Put the processed sand into a pan and heat it with strong fire until the sand becomes smooth and easy to be rotated. Add drugs in and stir – fry them together constantly to let the drugs covered by the sand. Take the drugs out when they swell, turn crisp in texture and yellow or deeper in color outside. Or put the drugs into vinegar for a short while when they are still hot, then take out for drying.

4. Amount of Adjuvant Material

The adjuvant material should cover the drug.

5. Suitable Drugs

Suitable drugs for this method are the drugs with hardy texture or toxicity.

6. Features

During processing, high temperature should be remained and the drugs should be stir – fired frequently. Take the drugs out and screen out the sand immediately when they are ready.

7. Notices

（1）Drugs should be dried before processing.

（2）Temperature should be controled.

（3）Remove the sand as quickly as possible after the drugs are taken out.

（4）Sometimes plant oil can be added into sand to make it smooth enough.

（5）The sand with oil can be used repeatedly.

Endothelium Corneum Gigeriae Galli（Jineijin）

【Source】Endothelium Corneum Gigeriae Galli is the dried inner wall of the gizzard of *Gallus gallus domesticus* Brisson（Fam. Phasianidae）.

【Processing Methods】

1. **Raw Endothelium Corneum Gigeriae Galli** Remove impurities, clean and dry the drugs.

2. **Stir – frying Endothelium Corneum Gigeriae Galli** Put the drugs in a hot pan, heat with medium fire and stir – fry them until the drugs turn coke yellow outside. Take it out and cool it down.

3. **Stir – frying Endothelium Corneum Gigeriae Galli with Sand** Put the sand into a pan and heat with medium fire until the sand becomes smooth. Add drugs which are cut into the same size and stir – fry them constantly until the drugs start to swell and curl. Take them out when the drugs become crisp and deep – yellow in color.

4. **Stir – frying Endothelium Corneum Gigeriae Galli with Vinegar** Crush the drugs and put them into a pan. Stir – fry the drugs quickly with mild fire until they swell. Then sprinkle vinegar on the drugs' surface and take them out, make them dry. Use 15kg vinegar for 100kg drugs.

Notices: Medium fire and river sand of medium size are the key factors for processing. Otherwise, the sand will be adhered to the drugs.

【Processing Functions】

1. Raw Endothelium Corneum Gigeriae Galli　The raw drug can remove stagnation, relieve stranguria and dissolve calculi. For example, it can be used in Shaling Pills. (Recorded in *Records of Chinese Medicine with Reference to Western Medicine*)

2. Stir – frying Endothelium Corneum Gigeriae Galli　Stir – frying can make the drug crisp in texture and easy to be crushed. And it's effects of fortifying the spleen and removing food stagnation are strengthened.

3. Stir – frying Endothelium Corneum Gigeriae Galli with Sand　Stir – frying with sand can also make the drug crisp in texture and easy to be crushed. Besides, the bad odor can be modified. The processed drug has the effects of soothing the liver and rectifying the spleen, and promoting urination.

【Processing Research】

The stir – fried drug has the functions of facilitating digestion and gastric emptying. When the drugs are stir – fried without adjuvant materials, the content of water, alcohol, and chloroform are the highest among all the processed products.

Semen Strychni (Maqianzi)

【Source】　Semen Strychni is the dried ripe seed of *Strychnos nux – vomica* L. (Fam. Loganiaceae).

【Processing Methods】

1. Raw Semen Strychni　Remove impurities and screen out ashes.

2. Stir – frying Semen Strychni with Sand　Put the sand into a hot pan, heat with strong fire until the sand becomes smooth. Add drugs in and stir – fry them together constantly until the drugs turn dark brown outside and bronzing inside. Take the drugs out when they expand with small bubbles on the surface.

3. Stir – frying Semen Strychni with Oil　Preheat the sesame oil to around 230℃ in a pan. Then put drugs in the oil and stir – fry them until the drugs become yellow.

4. Semen Strychni Pulveratum　Curara stir – fried with sand is crushed into a fine powder and mixed with suitable starch.

【Requirements】

1. The content of strychnine in raw drugs should be 1.20% ~ 2.20%.

2. The content of strychnine in Semen Strychni Pulveratum should be 0.78% ~ 0.82% and the moisture content less than 14%.

【Processing Functions】

1. Raw Semen Strychni　The raw drug is highly toxic and hard in texture, which is only for external uses.

2. Processed Semen Strychni　After being processed, the drug's toxicity is reduced. It becomes crisp in texture, which makes it easy to be crushed. It is proper for internal uses. It is usually used for wind – damp and arthralgia, injury, fracture and bruise, etc.

【Processing Research】

The content of strychnine will change when it is processed with different temperature, which would affect the toxicity and effectiveness of drugs. According to reports, the contents of strychnine in raw drugs, drugs stir – fried with sand, drugs stir – fried with oil, drugs stir – fried with urine and drugs stir – fried with vinegar are 1.975% , 1.970% , 1.980% , 0.389% and 0.374% respectively. Meanwhile, for the strychnine and vauqueline found in villus is far more less than those in seeds, the villus should be discarded before processing.

Stir – frying with Clam Powder

1. Definition

It is a method of stir – frying the cleaned or cut drugs with clam powder to a certain degree, normally with medium fire.

2. Amount of Adjuvant Material

Use 30 ~ 50kg clam powder for 100kg drugs.

3. Suitable Drugs

Suitable drugs are mastic drugs.

4. Notices

(1) Stir – fry the drugs separately according to their size.

(2) Do not use too strong fire while processing.

(3) Stir – fry drugs quickly and evenly in the pan.

(4) Change the adjuvant materials frequently.

(5) Use a few drugs to test the temperature before a great amount of valuable and slight drugs are being processed.

Colla Corii Asini (E'jiao)

【Source】 Colla Corii Asini is the solid glue prepared from the dried or fresh skin of *Equus asinus* Linnaeus (Fam. Equidae) by decoction and concentration.

【Processing Methods】

1. Raw Clump of Colla Corii Asini　Bake the bar of the drugs with mild fire until they become soft, then cut the drugs into small cubes.

2. Stir – frying Colla Corii Asini with clam powder　Put the clam powder into a hot pan and stir – fry with medium fire until they become smooth. Add the drugs in cubes in, stir – fry them together constantly until the drugs expand to a ball shape and have no hard parts but honeycomb – shape – like. Use 30 ~50kg clam powder per 100kg drugs.

3. Stir – frying Colla Corii Asini with Cattail Pollen　Put the Cattail Pollen into a hot pan and stir – fry them with medium fire until the color of the pollen changes slightly. Then add the cubes in and stir – fry them together constantly until the drugs expand to a ball shape and have no hard parts but honeycomb – shape – like inside.

【Processing Functions】

1. Raw Clump of Colla Corii Asini   The raw drug has the functions of tonifying the blood and enriching *yin*, which is often used for syndromes of deficiency of blood, sallow yellow, vigorous fire resulted from *yin* deficiency, vexation and insomnia. For example, it can be used in Huanglian Ejiao Decoction to treat cough caused by yin deficiency and insomnia (Recorded in *Treatise on Cold Damage and Miscellaneous Diseases*).

2. Stir – frying Colla Corii Asini with clam powder   The processing moderates the greasy nature of the drug, which makes it good at nourishing the lung and moistening the dryness. So it can be used for treating cough caused by *yin* deficiency. For example, it can be used in Bufei E'jiao Decoction to treat symptoms of deficiency of the lung and exuberant fire, cough, dry throat, and little phlegm (recorded in *Key to Diagnosis and Treatment of Children's Diseases*).

3. Stir – frying Colla Corii Asini with Cattail Pollen   This processing makes the drug have the function of stanching bleeding. For example, it can be used in Jiaoai Decoction to treat profuse uterine bleeding (recorded in *Synopsis of the Golden Chamber*) .

【Processing Research】

When the temperature of the clam powder is controled between 140℃ and 160℃ and the processing time is between 3 and 5 minutes, the drugs could have the best quality. The adjuvant materials should cover the drugs completely. And the drugs should be cut into the same size before processing and stir – fried continuously during processing.

Stir – frying with Talcum Powder

1. Definition

It is a method of stir – frying the cleaned or cut drugs with Talcum powder to a certain degree, normally with medium fire.

2. Amount of Adjuvant Material

Use 40 ~ 50kg Talcum powder for 100kg drugs.

3. Suitable Drugs

Suitable drugs are animal drugs with strong tenacity.

Cutis Erinacei (*Ciweipi*)

【Source】 Cutis Erinacei is the dried hide of *Erinaceus europaeus* L. or *Hemiehianus dauuricus* Sundevall (Fam. Erinaceidae) .

【Processing Methods】

1. Raw Cutis Erinacei　Soak the drugs in alkali water and brush to make them clean. Then moisten them thoroughly, cut drugs into small cubes, and dry them.

2. Stir－frying Cutis Erinacei with Talcum powder　Stir－fry the talcum powder in a preheated pan with medium fire until the powder becomes smooth. Put the cleaned drugs in cubes into the powder and stir－fry them quickly until the stingers are curled and bald. Use 40kg talcum powder per 100kg drugs.

【Processing Purposes】

1. Remove the bad odor and taste.

2. Make the drugs loose in texture and easy to be decocted.

Other drugs

Types	Drugs	Processing Functions
Stir－frying with Wheat Bran	Rhizoma Atractylodis Macrocephala (*Baizhu*)	Moderate the nature of dryness and strengthen the functions of fortifying the spleen and relieving distention
	Rhizoma Dioscoreae (*Shanyao*)	Strengthen the function of fortifying the spleen and remove the bad odor
Stir－frying with Rice	Huechys (*Hongniangzi*)	Reduce toxicity
Stir－frying with Sand	Carapax et Plastrum Testudinis (*Guijia*)	Remove the bad odor and facilitate the grinding
	Carapax Trionycis (*Biejia*)	Facilitate the grinding
Stir－frying with Talc Powder	Hirudo (*Shuizhi*)	Reduce toxicity and facilitate the grinding

第八章　炒　法

1. 炒法的定义

将净制或切制过的药物置炒制容器内不断翻动或转动，或先将辅料加热，然后加入药物进行加工炮制的方法。

2. 炒法的种类

（1）清炒法

炒黄：用文火或中火加热，使药物表面呈黄色或颜色加深，或发泡鼓起，或爆裂，并逸出固有气味的方法。

炒焦：用中火或武火加热，炒至药物表面呈焦黄或焦褐色。

炒炭：用武火或中火加热，炒至药物表面焦黑色或焦褐色。

（2）加辅料炒法

可分为麦麸炒、米炒、土炒、砂炒、蛤粉炒和滑石粉炒等。

3. 炒制工艺

将净制或切制过的药物，筛去灰屑，大小分档，置预热过的炒制容器内，加辅料或不加辅料，用不同火力加热，并不断翻动或转动使之达到一定程度。

4. 炒法的操作

主要操作方法有手工炒和机器炒。手工炒制的优点是所需仪器简单，适合于小规模生产，而机器炒制则更适用于大规模生产。其操作要点如下：①炒制过程中翻炒迅速，炒好后快速出锅和翻动；②适合于加工炮制少量多种类的药物。

第一节　清炒法

一、炒黄

1. 定义

将净制或切制过的药物，置炒制容器内，用文火或中火加热，并不断翻动或转动，使药物表面呈黄色或颜色加深的方法。

2. 炒黄的目的

（1）增强疗效。
（2）降低毒性或副作用。

3. 工艺

将净制或切制过的药物，筛去灰屑，大小分档，置预热过的炒制容器内，不加辅料，用不同火力加热，并不断翻动或转动使之达到一定程度。

4. 判断标准

（1）断面呈淡黄色。
（2）颜色加深。
（3）有爆鸣声。
（4）外观形态改变（发泡鼓起）。
（5）爆裂。
（6）逸出固有气味。

5. 注意事项

当药物炒至淡黄色时，注意避免炒焦。通常使用文火加热，而对一些特殊药材可使用中火进行加热，如苍耳子、王不留行、牛蒡子以及薏苡仁等。

6. 适用药材

果实类与种子类药材适用炒黄法进行炮制，某些根茎类甚至是动物药也使用此法进行炮制，如赤芍、槐花、九香虫和海螵蛸。

芥　子

【来源】本品为十字花科植物白芥或芥的干燥成熟种子。

【炮制方法】

1. **芥子**　取原药材，去净杂质，用时捣碎。

2. **炒芥子**　取净芥子，置炒制容器内，用文火加热，炒至颜色加深，有爆鸣声，断面浅黄色，有香气逸出时即可。

【炮制作用】

1. **芥子**　辛散力强，善于通络止痛。多用于胸闷胁痛，关节疼痛，痈肿疮毒。

2. **炒芥子**　缓和辛散走窜之性，可避免耗气伤阴，并善于顺气豁痰。多用于痰多咳嗽，如三子养亲汤（《韩氏医通》）。

【炮制目的】

1. 缓和辛散走窜之性，避免耗气伤阴。

2. 利于粉碎和煎出。

3. 杀酶保苷。

4. 避免成分损失，保留有效成分。

5. 适用于不同的临床需求。

【炮制研究】

芥子主要含有硫苷化合物，主要为芥子苷，酶解后生成具有健胃化痰作用的异硫氰酸酯类（芥子油）。炒后可杀酶保苷，使其服用后，在胃肠道环境中缓慢分解，逐渐释放出芥子油而发挥止咳化痰作用。

酸 枣 仁

【来源】本品为鼠李科植物酸枣的干燥成熟种子。

【炮制方法】

1. **酸枣仁** 取原药材，去净杂质。用时捣碎。

2. **炒酸枣仁** 取净酸枣仁，置炒制容器内，用文火加热，炒至鼓起，颜色加深，有爆鸣声，断面浅黄色，有香气时取出。

【炮制作用】

1. **酸枣仁** 功善宁心安神，多用于心阴不足和肝肾亏损的惊悸，健忘，眩晕，虚烦不眠等症，如酸枣仁汤（《金匮要略》）。

2. **炒酸枣仁** 养心安神作用强于生酸枣仁，如治疗心虚血少之心悸健忘、失眠多梦的养心汤（《良方》）。

【炮制目的】

1. 酸枣仁炒后种皮开裂，易于粉碎和煎出。其有效成分含量为：①酸枣仁含量为16.2%；②炒酸枣仁含量为17.4%；③酸枣仁炭含量为13.8%。

2. 增强了镇静安神作用。

【炮制研究】

据报道，生、炒酸枣仁具有相同的功效，而炒炭品则失去了养心安神的功效。

牵 牛 子

【来源】本品为旋花科植物裂叶牵牛或圆叶牵牛的干燥成熟种子。

【炮制方法】

1. **牵牛子** 取原药材，去净杂质，用时捣碎。

2. **炒牵牛子** 取净牵牛子，置炒制容器内，用文火加热，炒至膨胀鼓起，有爆裂声，颜色加深，断面浅黄色，逸出香气时即可。

【炮制作用】

1. **牵牛子** 具有泻水通便，消痰涤饮，杀虫攻积的功能，如用于治水肿胀满的舟车丸（《景岳》）。

2. **炒牵牛子** 多用于食积不化，气逆痰壅。如治小儿停乳停食，腹胀便秘，痰盛喘咳的一捻金（《中国药典》）。

【炮制目的】

1. 降低毒性，缓和药性。

2. 使药物质地酥脆，易于有效成分的溶出。

3. 适用于不同的临床需求。

【炮制研究】

牵牛子中含有牵牛子苷和生物碱。牵牛子苷具有刺激肠道，增加肠蠕动的作用。经过炒制后，牵牛子苷含量减少，缓和了泻水通便的作用。

苍 耳 子

【来源】本品为菊科植物苍耳的干燥成熟带总苞的果实。

【炮制方法】

1. **苍耳子** 取原药材，除去杂质，用时捣碎。

2. **炒苍耳子** 取净苍耳子，置炒制容器内，用中火加热，炒至焦黄色，刺焦时即可，碾去刺，筛净。

【炮制作用】

1. **苍耳子** 散风湿，止痒。

2. **炒苍耳子** 降低毒性，偏于通鼻窍，驱风湿，止痛。

【炮制目的】

1. 降低毒性。

2. 易于除刺。

【炮制研究】

苍耳子在经过炒制之后，其所含的毒性成分会发生变性而使毒性降低，与此同时，由于炒制过程中使用中火加热，可使苍耳刺易于除去，有效成分相对含量增加，从而提高了药物的疗效。

莱 菔 子

【来源】本品为十字花科植物萝卜的干燥成熟种子。

【炮制方法】

1. **莱菔子** 取原药材，去净杂质，用时捣碎。

2. **炒莱菔子** 取净莱菔子，置炒制容器内，用文火加热，炒至鼓起，鸣爆声减弱，手拈易碎，断面浅黄色，有香气逸出时即可。

【炮制作用】

1. **莱菔子** 能升能散，长于涌吐风痰。

2. **炒莱菔子** 炒后变升为降，长于消食除胀、降气化痰。如治疗气喘咳嗽的三子养亲汤（《保元》）；治疗食积不化的保和丸（《中国药典》）。

【炮制目的】

1. 缓和药性，消除毒副作用。

2. 易于粉碎和煎出，提高疗效。

薏 苡 仁

【来源】本品为禾本科植物薏苡的干燥成熟种仁。

【炮制方法】

1. **薏苡仁**　取原药材，除去杂质，筛去灰屑。

2. **炒薏苡仁**　取净薏苡仁，置炒制容器内，用中火加热，炒至表面黄色，略鼓起，表面有突起，取出。

3. **麸炒薏苡仁**　先将锅烧热，撒入麦麸即刻烟起，再投入薏苡仁迅速拌炒至黄色，微鼓起，取出，筛去麦麸即得。每100kg薏苡仁，用麦麸15kg。

【炮制作用】

1. **薏苡仁**　性寒凉，长于利水渗湿，清热排脓，除弊止痛。

2. **炮制品**　缓和生品寒凉之性，长于健脾止泻，可用于脾虚泄泻，纳少腹胀。如参苓白术散（《中国药典》）。

王 不 留 行

【来源】本品为石竹科植物麦蓝菜的干燥成熟种子。

【炮制方法】

1. **王不留行**　取原药材，去净杂质，洗净，干燥。

2. **炒王不留行**　取净王不留行，投入已用中火烧热的锅内，迅速拌炒至大部分爆花即可。

【炮制作用】

1. **王不留行**　长于消痈肿，用于乳痈或其他疮痈肿痛，如王不留行散（《医心方》）。

2. **炒王不留行**　质地松泡，利于有效成分煎出，长于活血通经，下乳，通淋，如用于通乳四物汤（《医略六书》）。

【炮制目的】

1. 使有效成分易于煎出。

2. 扩大药用范围。

【炮制研究】

王不留行的功效与其有效成分的溶出率密切相关，而溶出物的增加与炒制程度和爆花程度有关。在炒至生品，未爆花，刚爆花与完全爆花时，其水溶物含量分别为7.11%，8.58%，11.56%和14.39%；当炒制品爆花率为60%，70%，80%，90%和100%时，其溶出率分别为11.69%，12.36%，13.11%，13.80%和14.39%。爆花率越高，溶出率越高。

二、炒焦

1. 定义

将净选或切制后的药物，置炒制容器内，用中火或武火加热。

2. 炒焦的目的

（1）增强药物消食健脾的功效，如麦芽、谷芽和神曲。

（2）减少药物的刺激性，如槟榔、栀子和川楝子。

3. 工艺

将净制或切制过的药物，筛去灰屑，大小分档，置预热过的炒制容器内，不加辅料，用不同火力加热，并不断翻动或转动使之达到一定程度。

4. 判断标准

（1）药物表面呈焦黄或焦褐色，内部焦黄，如山楂和神曲。

（2）药物表面呈焦黄色，内部颜色加深，如山楂和谷芽。

5. 注意事项

当炒焦药物时，注意避免炭化。

6. 适用药物

适用炒焦法进行炮制的药物多具健脾养胃之功效，对肠胃造成刺激的药物也可用此法进行炮制。

栀　　子

【来源】本品为茜草科植物栀子的干燥成熟果实。

【炮制方法】

1. **栀子**　取原药材，除去杂质，碾碎。

2. **炒栀子**　取栀子碎块，置炒制容器内，用文火加热，炒至深黄色。

3. **焦栀子**　取栀子碎块，置炒制容器内，用中火加热，炒至焦黄色。

4. **栀子炭**　取栀子碎块，置炒制容器内，用武火加热炒至黑褐色，喷淋少许清水熄灭火星。

【炮制作用】

1. **栀子**　味苦，性寒，长于泻火利湿，凉血解毒。如治温病高热烦躁，神昏谵语的栀子仁汤（《不居集》），治湿热黄疸的茵陈蒿汤（《伤寒》），治跌打损伤，青肿疼痛，可用栀子研末与面粉、黄酒调敷。

2. **焦栀子**　缓和苦寒之性，具有清热除烦的功用。

3. **栀子炭**　微有苦寒之性，善于凉血止血，如十灰散（《十药》）。

【炮制目的】

1. 产生新功效，增强原有功效。

2. 缓和药性。

【炮制研究】

栀子尚有其他炮制方法，如用姜汁制，去皮等。无论采用何种炮制方法，京尼平苷和熊果酸的含量都会减少，因此其药理作用会受到影响和改变。例如，栀子在利胆、止血、退热、抑菌等方面的作用因其炮制方法的不同而不同，其中，镇静和止血作用以焦栀子为最佳。

山　楂

【来源】本品为蔷薇科植物山里红或山楂的干燥成熟果实。

【炮制方法】

1. **山楂**　取原药材，除去杂质及脱落的核及果柄。

2. **炒山楂**　取净山楂，置炒制容器内，用中火加热，炒至颜色加深。

3. **焦山楂**　取净山楂，置炒制容器内，用中火加热，炒至外表焦褐色，内部焦黄色。

4. **山楂炭**　取净山楂，置炒制容器内，用武火加热，炒至表面焦黑色，内部焦褐色。

【炮制作用】

1. **山楂**　长于活血化瘀。

2. **炒山楂**　酸味减弱，可缓和对胃的刺激性，善于消食化积。用于脾虚食滞，食欲不振，神倦乏力。

3. **焦山楂**　不仅酸味减弱，且增加了苦味，长于消食止泻。用于食积兼脾虚和痢疾，如治疗饮食积滞的保和丸（《中国药典》）。

4. **山楂炭**　其性收涩，具有止血、止泻的功效。

【炮制研究】

山楂生品中有机酸含量最高，炒制品其次，焦山楂中含量最低，炮制品中有机酸含量降低了68%。生山楂与炒山楂较之其他炮制品具有更强的促进消化能力，而生山楂和焦山楂较之其他炮制品具有更强的抑菌作用。

槟　榔

【来源】本品为棕榈科植物槟榔的干燥成熟种子。

【炮制方法】

1. **槟榔**　取原药材，润透，切薄片，干燥。

2. **炒槟榔**　取槟榔片，置炒制容器内，用文火加热，炒至微黄色。

3. **焦槟榔**　取槟榔片，置炒制容器内，用中火加热，炒至焦黄色。

4. **槟榔炭**　取槟榔片，置炒制容器内，用武火加热，炒至焦黑色。

【炮制作用】

1. **槟榔**　具有杀虫，消积，降气，行水，截疟的功能。

2. **炒槟榔**　缓和药性，减少副作用，长于消食导滞。

3. **焦槟榔**　缓和药性，增强消食导滞之功效，如治疗饮食停滞、腹中胀痛的开胸顺气丸（《中成药制剂手册》）。

4. **槟榔炭**　长于止血。

【炮制目的】

1. 增强疗效，缓和药性。

2. 适用于更多的临床需求。

【炮制研究】

炮制槟榔时，采用"少泡多润"的原则可避免药物有效成分的流失。研究显示，槟榔生品和炒制品中槟榔碱的含量分别为 0.4% ~ 0.52% 和 0.13% ~ 0.31%。经过浸泡之后，生物碱含量降低 24% ，而使其杀虫功效减弱。同时，应在阴凉通风处对饮片进行干燥，槟榔炒炭时温度不宜过高。

三、炒炭

1. 定义

用武火或中火加热药物炒至其炭化。

2. 炒炭的目的

（1）增强或产生止血作用，如地榆和蒲黄。
（2）增强药物的止泻作用，如乌梅炭和石榴皮炭。

3. 工艺

将净制或切制过的药物，筛去灰屑，大小分档，置预热过的炒制容器内，不加辅料，用不同火力加热，并不断翻动或转动使之达到一定程度，并喷淋少许清水灭尽火星。

4. 判断标准

（1）炒至药物表面焦黑色或焦褐色，如根与块茎类药物。
（2）达到"炒炭存性"要求，如花、叶和全草类药物。
（3）药物表面呈黑色且具有光泽，如茜草等。

5. 注意事项

（1）操作时要掌握好火力，质地坚实的药物宜用武火，质地疏松的花、花粉、叶、全草类药物可用中火，视具体药物灵活掌握。
（2）需喷淋适量清水灭尽火星，以免引起燃烧。
（3）炒炭要求存性。
（4）药物必须在晾凉之后贮藏，避免复燃。

6. 适用药物

此法适用于具有止血、止泻作用的药物。

地　　榆

【来源】本品为蔷薇科植物地榆或长叶地榆的干燥根。
【炮制方法】
1. **地榆**　取原药材，除去旁枝，切厚片。
2. **地榆炭**　取地榆片，置于用武火预热过的炒制容器内，快速炒至表面焦黑色，内部棕褐色。

【炮制作用】

1. **地榆**　凉血，解毒，止痛。

2. **地榆炭**　长于收敛止血，如用于治疗烧烫伤。

【炮制目的】

1. 增强止血之功效。

2. 适用于更多的临床需求。

【炮制研究】

经过炒炭之后，地榆具有止血和抑菌的药理作用，可用于治疗烧烫伤。

干　姜

【来源】本品为姜科植物姜的干燥根茎。

【炮制方法】

1. **干姜**　取原药材，除去杂质，切厚片或块。

2. **炮姜**　先将净河砂置炒制容器内，用武火炒热，再加入干姜片或块，不断翻动，炒至鼓起，表面棕褐色。

3. **姜炭**　取干姜块，置炒制容器内，用武火加热，炒至表面焦黑色，内部棕褐色，喷淋少许清水，灭尽火星。

注意事项：炮制过程中保持通风，炒至无烟，并迅速晾凉。

【炮制作用】

1. **干姜**　味辛，性热。具有温中散寒、回阳通脉、燥湿消痰的功能。

2. **炮姜**　辛燥之性较干姜弱，长于温经止血。

3. **姜炭**　味苦、涩，性温。具有温中散寒、温经止血的功能，可用于附子理中丸与治疗血崩的如圣散（《丹溪》）等。

【炮制目的】

1. 有效成分更易溶出。

2. 适用于更多的临床需求。

【炮制研究】

对干姜、炮姜、姜炭的挥发油含量进行比较，结果表明，干姜含量最高；炮姜含量明显下降；姜炭含量最低，其炮制品长于治疗溃疡与止血。

蒲　黄

【来源】本品为香蒲科植物水烛香蒲、东方香蒲或同属植物的干燥花粉。

【炮制方法】

1. **蒲黄**　取原药材，揉碎结块，除去花丝及杂质。

2. **蒲黄炭**　取净蒲黄，置炒制容器内，用中火加热，炒至棕褐色，喷淋少许清水，灭尽火星。

注意事项：炒制时火力不可过大以免灰化，检查确已凉透后方能贮藏。

【炮制作用】

1. 蒲黄　味甘，性平，具有行血化瘀，止痛的功能，可用于少腹逐瘀汤。

2. 蒲黄炭　性涩，止血作用增强，可用于四红片。

【炮制目的】

蒲黄生品具有促进血液循环之功效，炭品功擅止血，可见炮制的首要作用是改变了药物的性质，另外也改变了临床应用。

【炮制研究】

蒲黄炭品较之生品有更强的抑制溶纤维蛋白酶的作用，药理学试验表明，炭品能缩短小鼠的凝血时间，说明炒炭保证了止血的功效。

第二节　加辅料炒法

一、麸炒

1. 定义

将净制或切制后的药物用麦麸熏炒至一定程度的方法，通常使用中火炒制。

2. 麸炒的目的

（1）降低挥发油的含量。

（2）加热药物。

（3）使炮制过程有充足的时间或热量。

（4）矫臭矫味。

（5）增强药物补气和中、涩肠止泻之功效。

3. 工艺

先用中火或武火将锅烧热，再将麦麸均匀撒入热锅中，至起烟时投入药物，快速均匀翻动，炒至药物表面呈黄色，麦麸变黑时取出。

4. 辅料用量

每100kg 药物，用麦麸 10～15kg。

5. 适用药物

常用麦麸炒制补脾胃或作用强烈及有腥味的药物。

6. 注意事项

（1）使用中火对锅进行预热。

（2）麦麸要均匀撒布热锅中。

（3）麸炒药物要求干燥。

（4）麸炒药物达到标准时要求迅速出锅。

枳　壳

【来源】本品为芸香科植物酸橙的干燥未成熟果实。

【炮制方法】

1. **枳壳**　取原药材，除去杂质，洗净，润透，去核，切薄片，色黄白，气芳香。

2. **麸炒枳壳**　先将锅烧热，均匀撒入定量麦麸，用中火加热，待烟起投入枳壳片，不断翻动，炒至淡黄色，麦麸变黑时取出。每 100kg 枳壳片，用麦麸 10kg。

【炮制作用】

1. **枳壳**　辛燥，长于行气宽中除胀，如用于血府逐瘀汤。

2. **麸炒枳壳**　缓和其峻烈之性，长于理气健胃消食，如治积滞内停，胃脘痞满的木香槟榔丸（《局方》）。

【炮制目的】

1. 缓和药性。

2. 扩大临床药用范围。

【炮制研究】

枳壳麸炒之后挥发油含量降低，缓和了其峻烈之性并增强了健胃的功效。因为大部分挥发油和药效成分存在于枳壳的皮中，应去掉几乎不含有效成分的果肉部分。

苍　术

【来源】本品为菊科植物茅苍术或北苍术的干燥根茎。

【炮制方法】

1. **苍术**　取原药材，除去杂质，用水浸泡，洗净，润透，切厚片。

2. **麸炒苍术**　先将锅烧热，撒入麦麸，用中火加热，待冒烟时投入苍术片，不断翻炒至深黄色时，取出。每 100kg 苍术片，用麦麸 10kg。

3. **焦苍术**　取苍术片置热锅内，用中火加热，炒至焦褐色时即可。

【炮制作用】

1. **苍术**　祛风除湿散寒，用于风湿痹痛。如治风湿痹痛的薏苡仁汤（《治裁》）。

2. **麸炒苍术**　辛性减弱，燥性缓和，气变芳香，增强了健脾和胃的作用。

3. **焦苍术**　辛燥之性大减，以固肠止泻为主。如治脾虚泄泻的椒术丸（《保命集》）。

【炮制研究】

苍术挥发油中的主要成分为苍术醇和苍术酮。经过麸炒之后，苍术醇和苍术酮的含量明显减少，起到了缓和“燥性”的作用。

僵　蚕

【来源】本品为蚕蛾科昆虫家蚕 4～5 龄的幼虫感染（或人工接种）白僵菌而致死的干燥体。

【炮制方法】

1. **僵蚕**　取原药材，除去杂质及残丝，洗净，晒干。

2. 麸炒僵蚕 先用中火将锅烧热，均匀撒入定量麦麸，待起烟时加入净僵蚕，急速翻炒至表面呈黄色时出锅。每 100kg 僵蚕，用麦麸 10kg。

【炮制作用】

1. 僵蚕 长于祛风定惊、化痰散结，可用于治疗风热所引发的头痛等症。

2. 麸炒僵蚕 长于化痰散结，用于瘰疬痰核，中风失音。如治喉风，咽喉肿痛的白僵蚕散（《魏氏家藏方》）。

【炮制目的】

1. 净制药物。

2. 保持或增强疗效。

3. 矫臭矫味，便于服用。

4. 去除表面微生物。

二、米炒

1. 定义

将净制或切制后的药物与米同炒至一定程度的方法，一般使用中火加热。

2. 功能

（1）指示炮制程度。

（2）加热药物。

（3）吸附药物的毒性成分。

（4）增强药物的健脾止泻作用。

3. 工艺

先将锅烧热，加入定量的米，用中火炒至冒烟时，投入药物，快速拌炒至药物表面颜色加深，米呈焦黄或焦褐色，取出。

4. 辅料用量

每 100kg 药物，用米 20kg。

5. 适用药物

毒性药物（斑蝥）和具有补脾益气作用的药物（党参）。

6. 注意事项

（1）炮制昆虫类药物时，一般以米的色泽观察火候。

（2）炮制植物类药物时，观察药物色泽变化。

党 参

【来源】本品为桔梗科植物党参、素花党参或川党参的干燥根。

【炮制方法】

1. **党参** 取原药材，除去杂质，洗净，润透，切厚片。

2. **米炒党参** 将大米置热的炒药锅内，用中火加热至米冒烟时，投入党参片拌炒，至党参呈黄色时取出。每100kg党参片，用米20kg。

3. **蜜炙党参** 取炼蜜用适量开水稀释后，与党参片拌匀，闷透，置热炒药锅内，用文火加热，不断翻炒至黄棕色，不黏手时取出。每100kg党参片，用炼蜜20kg。

【炮制作用】

1. **党参** 擅长益气生津，如治气阴两亏的上党参膏（《得配》）；治气血两亏的两仪膏（《中药成方集》）。

2. **米炒党参** 气变清香，增强了和胃、健脾止泻的作用。如具补中益气之功的参芪白术汤；治脾虚泄泻的理中汤（《伤寒论》）。

3. **蜜炙党参** 增强了补中益气，润燥养阴的作用。

【炮制研究】

研究表明，党参入药以厚片为宜，有利于药效成分煎出。

斑　蝥

【来源】本品为芫青科昆虫南方大斑蝥或黄黑小斑蝥的干燥体。

【炮制方法】

1. **斑蝥** 取原药材，除去头、足、翅及杂质。

2. **米炒斑蝥** 将米置热锅中，用中火加热至冒烟，投入斑蝥拌炒，至米呈黄棕色，取出。每100kg斑蝥，用米20kg。

【炮制作用】

1. **斑蝥** 长于攻毒蚀疮，用于治疗痈疽肿毒。

2. **米炒斑蝥** 以通经、破癥散结为主，如治淤血阻滞、月经闭塞的斑蝥通经丸（《济阴》）。

【炮制目的】

1. 降低毒性，增强疗效。

2. 米可用于指示炮制程度。

【炮制研究】

斑蝥中的有毒物质为斑蝥素，其在84℃开始升华，升华点为110℃。米炒时锅温为128℃，正适合于斑蝥素的升华。当斑蝥与米同炒时，由于斑蝥均匀受热，使斑蝥素部分升华而含量降低，从而使其毒性降低。

加热过程中，要注意避免温度过高而引起炭化，注意通风以避免吸入有毒成分，加工净制斑蝥之后要立即洗净双手。

三、土炒

1. 定义

将净制或切制后的药物与灶心土同炒至一定程度的方法，一般使用中火加热。

2. 功能

能增强补脾止泻的功能。

3. 工艺

将灶心土研成细粉，置于锅内，用中火加热，炒至土呈灵活状态时投入净药物，翻炒至药物表面均匀挂上一层土粉，并透出香气时，取出，筛去土粉。

4. 辅料用量

每100kg 药物，用土粉 25～30kg。

5. 适用药物

具有补脾止泻功能的药物。

白　术

【来源】本品为菊科植物白术的干燥根茎。

【炮制方法】

1. **白术**　取原药材，除去杂质，用水洗净，润透，切厚片。

2. **土炒白术**　先将土置锅内，用中火加热，炒至土呈灵活状态时，投入白术片，炒至白术表面均匀挂上土粉时，取出。每100kg 白术片，用灶心土 25kg。

3. **麸炒白术**　先将锅用中火烧热，撒入麦麸，待冒烟时，投入白术片，不断翻炒，至白术呈焦黄色，逸出焦香气，取出。每100kg 白术片，用麦麸 10kg。

【炮制作用】

1. **白术**　健脾燥湿，利水消肿。

2. **土炒白术**　借土气助脾，补脾止泻力胜。

3. **麸炒白术**　缓和燥性，借麸入中，增强健脾、消胀作用。

【炮制目的】

1. 缓和药物燥性。

2. 扩大临床药用范围。

3. 增强药物疗效。

【炮制研究】

白术经过炮制后挥发油含量有所减少，缓和了药物的燥性。

山　药

【来源】本品为薯蓣科植物薯蓣的干燥根茎。

【炮制方法】

1. **山药**　取原药材，除去杂质，大小分开，洗净，润透，切厚片。

2. **土炒山药**　先将土粉置锅内，用中火加热至灵活状态，再投入山药片拌炒，至表面均匀挂土粉时，取出。每100kg 山药片，用灶心土 30kg。

3. **麸炒山药** 将锅烧热，撒入麦麸，待其冒烟时，投入山药片，用中火加热，不断翻动至黄色，并逸出焦香气时，取出。每 100kg 山药片，用麦麸 10kg。

【炮制作用】

1. **山药** 以补肾生精，益肺阴为主，如用于六味地黄丸。

2. **土炒山药** 以补脾止泻为主。

3. **麸炒山药** 以补脾健胃为主。

【炮制研究】

通过对山药、清炒山药、土炒山药和麸炒山药中薯蓣皂苷元的含量测定，发现其含量分别为11.69%，12.36%，13.11%和13.80%，表明山药经过炮制之后，其有效成分含量增加，因而提高了药效。

春季或秋季最适宜对山药进行加工处理，要即使干燥药材避免发生腐烂。炮制辅料用土需经常更换以保证疗效。

四、砂炒

1. 定义

将净制或切制后的药物与热砂用武火加热，同炒至一定程度的方法。

2. 功能

（1）便于调剂和制剂。

（2）便于去毛。

（3）降低毒性。

（4）矫臭矫味。

3. 工艺

取制过的砂置锅内，用武火加热至灵活状态，容易翻动时，投入药物，不断用砂掩埋，翻动，至质地酥脆或鼓起，外表呈黄色或较原色加深时，取出，或趁热投入醋中略浸，取出，干燥即得。

4. 辅料用量

以能掩盖所加药物为度。

5. 适用药物

适用于质地坚硬或具有毒性的药物。

6. 特点

炮制过程中应保持高温，翻动要勤，成品出锅要快并迅速筛去砂。

7. 注意事项

（1）药物在炮制之前需经干燥处理。

（2）砂炒温度要适中。

（3）出锅后尽快出去砂。

（4）有时可在砂中加入植物油使其更加灵活。

（5）油砂可反复使用。

鸡　内　金

【来源】本品为雉科动物家鸡的干燥沙囊内壁。

【炮制方法】

1. **鸡内金**　取原药材，除去杂质，洗净，干燥。

2. **炒鸡内金**　将净鸡内金置热锅内，用中火加热，炒至表面焦黄色，取出，放凉。

3. **砂炒鸡内金**　取砂子置锅内，用中火加热至灵活状态，投入大小一致的鸡内金，不断翻动，炒至鼓起卷曲、酥脆、呈深黄色时取出。

4. **醋鸡内金**　将鸡内金压碎，置锅内用文火加热，炒至鼓起，喷醋，取出，干燥。每100kg鸡内金，用醋15kg。

注意事项：砂炒鸡内金宜用中火，选用中粗河砂进行炒制，否则成品会出现黏砂现象。

【炮制作用】

1. **鸡内金**　长于攻积，通淋化石，如治砂石淋证的砂淋丸（《参西录》）。

2. **炒鸡内金**　质地酥脆，便于粉碎，并增强健脾消积的作用。

3. **砂炒鸡内金**　质地酥脆，便于粉碎，并改善其臭味，具有疏肝助脾，利尿通淋之功效。

【炮制研究】

鸡内金炒制之后具有助消化作用，能使胃排空速率加快。鸡内金经过清炒后，水、乙醇和氯仿浸出物含量在各炮制品中均为最高。

马　钱　子

【来源】本品为马钱子科植物马钱的干燥成熟种子。

【炮制方法】

1. **马钱子**　取原药材，除去杂质，筛去灰屑。

2. **砂烫马钱子**　将砂置热锅内，用武火加热至灵活状态，投入大小一致的马钱子，不断翻动，至棕褐色，鼓起，内部红褐色，并起小泡时，取出。

3. **油炸马钱子**　取麻油适量置锅内，加热至230℃左右，投入马钱子，炸至老黄色时，取出。

4. **马钱子粉**　取砂烫马钱子，粉碎成细粉，并加入适量淀粉。

【质量要求】

1. 生马钱子按干燥品计算，含士的宁应为1.20%~2.20%。

2. 马钱子粉按干燥品计算，含士的宁应为0.78%~0.82%，水分不得过14%。

【炮制作用】

1. **马钱子**　毒性剧烈，质地坚硬，仅供外用。

2. 制马钱子　毒性降低，质地酥脆，易于粉碎，可供内服。多用于风湿痹痛，跌打损伤，骨折瘀痛等。

【炮制研究】

马钱子炮制因受热程度的不同，其士的宁含量也不同，因而加工程度会影响药物的毒性和有效性。文献报道，马钱子生品、砂烫品、油炸品、尿泡品和醋淬品中士的宁含量分别为 1.975%，1.970%，1.980%，0.389% 和 0.374%。同时，马钱子皮毛中士的宁和马钱子碱含量均远低于种子中，因此马钱子在炮制之前需要去毛。

五、蛤粉炒

1. 定义

将净制或切制后的药物与蛤粉用中火加热，同炒至一定程度的方法。

2. 辅料用量

每 100kg 药物，用蛤粉 30～50kg。

3. 适用药物

胶类药物。

4. 注意事项

（1）药物需大小分档，分别炒制。

（2）炒制时火力不宜过大。

（3）胶丁下锅翻炒要速度快而均匀。

（4）辅料需经常更换。

（5）贵重、细料药物在大批炒制前采取试投的方法，以便掌握火力，保证炒制品质量。

阿　　胶

【来源】本品为马科动物驴的皮经煎煮、浓缩制成的固体胶。

【炮制方法】

1. 阿胶丁　取阿胶块，置文火上烘软，切成小丁块。

2. 蛤粉炒阿胶　取蛤粉适量置热锅内，用中火加热炒至灵活状态，投入阿胶丁，不断翻动，炒至鼓起呈圆球形，内无溏心时取出。每 100kg 阿胶丁，用蛤粉 30～50kg。

3. 蒲黄炒阿胶　将蒲黄置热锅内，用中火加热炒至稍微变色，投入阿胶丁，不断翻动，炒至鼓起呈圆球形，内无溏心时取出。

【炮制作用】

1. 阿胶丁　具有补血滋阴的功效，用于血虚萎黄，如用治阴虚火旺、心烦失眠的黄连阿胶汤（《伤寒》）。

2. 蛤粉炒阿胶　降低了滋腻之性，善于益肺润燥，用于阴虚咳嗽。如治肺虚火盛，咳喘咽干痰少的补肺阿胶汤 (《药证》)。

3. 蒲黄炒阿胶 以止血安络力胜，如用治冲任不固，崩中漏下，妊娠下血的胶艾汤 (《金匮》)。

【炮制研究】

蛤粉温度在 140℃ ~ 160℃ 之间，时间在 3 ~ 5 分钟时，炮制品质量较好。炮制时辅料应完全盖过药物表面，炒制之前应将药物切成统一大小，炒制过程中要注意不断翻动药物。

六、滑石粉炒

1. 定义

将净制或切制后的药物与滑石粉用中火加热，同炒至一定程度的方法。

2. 辅料的用量

每 100kg 药物，用蛤粉 40 ~ 50kg。

3. 适用药物

韧性较大的动物类药物。

<h1 style="text-align:center">刺 猬 皮</h1>

【来源】本品为猬科动物刺猬或短刺猬的干燥皮。

【炮制方法】

1. 刺猬皮 取原药材，用碱水浸泡，将污垢洗刷干净，再用清水洗净，润透，剁成小方块，干燥。

2. 滑石粉炒刺猬皮 取滑石粉置热锅中，用中火加热炒至灵活状态，投入净刺猬皮块，拌炒至黄色、鼓起、皮卷曲、刺尖秃时，取出。每 100kg 刺猬皮，用滑石粉 40kg。

【炮制目的】

1. 矫臭矫味。

2. 使药物质地疏松，易于煎煮。

其他药物

种类	药物	炮制作用
麸炒	白术	缓和燥性，增强健脾消胀作用
	山药	增强健脾之功，除去不良气味
米炒	红娘子	降低毒性
砂炒	龟甲	矫臭矫味，易于粉碎
	鳖甲	易于粉碎
滑石粉炒	水蛭	降低毒性，易于粉碎

Chapter Nine
Stir – frying with Liquid Adjuvant Materials

1. Definition

Stir – frying with liquid adjuvant materials refers to the processing method that stir – fries purified or cut drugs with some liquid adjuvant materials, and infiltrates the adjuvant material into the drugs' interior.

2. Types

There are six types of liquid supplemental materials which are wine, vinegar, salt – water, ginger juice, honey and oil.

3. Differences between Stir - frying with Liquid and Solid Adjuvant Materials

In some aspects, there are differences between stir – frying with solid adjuvant materials and liquid adjuvant materials. The differences are as follows:

Aspects	Liquid Adjuvant Materials	Solid Adjuvant Materials
Temperature	Low	Medium or high
Time	Long	Short
Process	Adjuvant materials penetrating into drugs	Adjuvant materials not penetrating into drugs
Nature	Adjuvant materials make most drugs' physico – chemical properties change	As heat transfer, adjuvant materials strengthen effects and deepen the superficial color of drugs
Operation	Fry drugs first, then add adjuvant materials or evenly mix adjuvant materials with drugs first, then fry	Heat the adjuvant materials first, then add drugs

4. Classification

According to different adjuvant materials, stir – frying method could be classified into the following concrete methods, i. e. , stir – frying with wine, such as Radix et Rhizoma Rhei

(*Dahuang*) ; stir－frying with vinegar, such as Radix Kansui (*Gansui*) ; stir－frying with salt water, such as Cortex Phellodendri Chinensis (*Huangbo*) ; stir－frying with ginger juice, such as Cortex Magnoliae Officinalis (*Houpo*) ; stir－frying with refined honey, such as Herba Ephedrae (*Mahuang*) ; and stir－frying with oil, such as Radix Notoginseng (*Sanqi*) .

Section One　Stir－frying with Wine

1. Definition

Stir－frying with wine refers to the processing method that stir－fries purified or cut drugs with a certain amount of wine, and stir－fries them with mild fire to a certain degree.

2. Purposes

(1) Change drugs' properties. For example, the main effects of Radix Gentianae (*Longdan*) are to clear heat, purge fire and dry dampness. But after being stir－fried with wine, the main effects are changed to treat headache, swelling and pain of eye due to the pathogenic fire of the liver and gallbladder.

(2) Synergistic effect. After being processed, the drugs' effect of promoting blood flow to unblock collateral will be strengthened, such as Radix Angelicae Sinensis (*Danggui*) .

(3) Moderate drugs' properties. After being processed, the cold property of some drugs will be moderated, such as Rhizoma Coptidis (*Huanglian*) .

(4) Increase the dissolution rate of the effective components of drugs. After being processed, the dissolution rate of the effective components would be increased, the effect will be improved, such as Radix Scutellariae (*Huangqin*) .

(5) Modify smell and stink of some drugs. After being processed, the bad smell and stink of some animal drugs will be removed or reduced, such as Zaocys (*Wushaoshe*) .

(6) Reduce drugs' toxicity or side－effects, and make their texture become crisp and easy to be crushed, such as Venenum Bufonis (*Chansu*) .

3. Technology

There are two kinds of processing technologies.

(1) Mix wine with drugs firstly and then fry. The way is suitable for most drugs, especially for drugs with hard texture tuber.

Mix the cleaned or cut drugs with wine evenly until they are slightly moistened, put the drugs into a frying container after the wine is absorbed thoroughly, then fry with a mild fire until the drugs become dry.

(2) Fry drugs firstly and then sprinkle wine on the drugs' surface. The way is suitable for those drugs with crisp texture, such as Faeces Togopteri (*Wulingzhi*) .

Put the cleaned or cut drugs into a frying container, and heat it to some degree, then spray some wine evenly on the drugs' surface and fry them to make them dry.

4. Amount of Adjuvant Material

The amount of the liquid adjuvant material needed in the procedures of stir – frying with wine is 10 ~ 20kg yellow wine per 100kg drugs.

5. Suitable Drugs

(1) Suitable for drugs with bitter and cold nature, such as Radix et Rhizoma Rhei (*Dahuang*).

(2) Suitable for drugs with the effect of promoting blood flow to eliminate blood stasis, such as Radix Angelicae Sinensis (*Danggui*).

(3) Suitable for drugs with the effect of expelling wind and removing collaterals, such as Radix Clematidis (*Weilingxian*).

Rhizoma Coptidis (Huanglian)

【Source】 Rhizoma Coptidis is the dried rhizome of *Coptis chinensis* Franch. , *Coptis deltoidea* C. Y. Cheng et Hsiao or *Coptis teeta* Wall. (Fam. Ranunculaceae).

【Processing Methods】

1. **Raw Rhizoma Coptidis**　Take the raw drugs, remove impurities, wash quickly, moisten thoroughly, and cut into thin slices.

2. **Stir – frying Rhizome Coptidis with wine**　It is to put the slices of the drugs and yellow wine together, mixing them thoroughly and covering tightly. After the wine is absorbed thoroughly by the drugs, pour the drugs into a preheated pan, fry quickly with a mild fire to make the drugs dry. The amount should be 12.5kg yellow wine per 100kg drugs.

3. **Stir – frying Rhizome Coptidis with Medicinal Evodia Fruit Juice**　It is to decoct some Fructus Evodiae (*Wuzhuyu*) with water, discarding the residues and getting the decoction. Then, put the drugs into decoction, mixing thoroughly, and make the slices moistened. After the decoction is absorbed, put the drugs into a frying container and fry them quickly with a mild fire till they become dry. The amount is usually 10kg medicinal Evodia Fruit per 100kg drugs.

4. **Stir – frying Rhizome Coptidis with ginger juice**　It is to mix the drug slices evenly with ginger juice and make them moistened slightly. After the ginger juice is absorbed thoroughly, put the drugs into a preheated pan and fry them quickly with a mild fire till the drugs become dry. The amount is 10kg ginger per 100kg drugs.

【Processing Functions】

1. **Raw Rhizoma Coptidis**　It is bitter in flavor and cold in nature, and has the effect of clearing heat, expelling damp and purging the heart fire. It could be used in Huanglian Jiedu Decoction, suitable for pyretic toxicity, and could be used in Xiexin Decoction, suitable for bleeding

due to blood – heat.

2. Rhizoma Coptidis stir – fried with wine   It can strengthen the effects and moderate its bitter flavor and cold nature. After being processed with wine, it can clear away pathogenic fire in upper energizer, and can be used to treat conjunctival congestion and swell, and oral ulceration.

3. Stir – frying Rhizoma Coptidis with Medicinal Evodia Fruit juice   It can moderate the bitter flavor and cold nature and strengthen the effects of treating liver depression transforming into fire, relieving stagnation of *qi*, removing damp – heat and clearing away stagnation fire in liver and gall bladder. It can be used to treat diarrhea due to damp – heat of Xianglian Pills.

4. Stir – frying Rhizoma Coptidis with ginger juice   It can clear away stomach heat and stop vomiting. It can be used in Banxia Xiexin Decoction, suitable for vomiting induced by gastric heat.

【Processing Research】

In order to avoid the loss of the effective components, the raw drugs should be washed quickly before being processed. It is inadvisable to overdose or take it for a long time because though the cold nature has been moderated after being processed, the drugs would still damage stomachs. Meanwhile, the dissolution rates of effective components would be different according to the different shapes. For example, the dissolution rates are 26.34%, 47.50%, 58.17% and 72.43% in section, strip, bulky powder and fine powder, respectively.

Radix et Rhizoma Rhei (Dahuang)

【Source】Radix et Rhizoma Rhei is the dried root and rhizome of *Rheum palmatum* L., *Rheum tanguticum* Maxim. ex Balf. or *Rheum of ficinale* Baill. (Fam. Polygonaceae).

【Processing Methods】

1. Raw Radix et Rhizoma Rhei   It should be purified, distinguished according to size, washed clean, and taken out from water. The drugs would then be cut into chunks after they are softened by sprinkling, exposed in the air so as to become dry or made dry with low heat.

2. Stir – frying Radix et Rhizoma Rhei with wine   Spray some yellow wine evenly on the drugs, mix them thoroughly and cover closely to make the drugs moistened. After the wine is absorbed thoroughly, put the drugs into a frying container and fry them with mild fire to become dry. The amount should be 10kg wine per 100kg drugs.

3. Steaming Radix et Rhizoma Rhei with wine   It is to mix the raw drugs evenly with some wine, moistening the drugs until the wine is absorbed completely. Then steam the drugs in a container till they become pitchy color both outside and inside. The amount should be 30kg wine per 100kg drugs.

4. Stir – frying Radix et Rhizoma Rhei with vinegar   It is to mix the raw drugs evenly with some vinegar, moistening the drugs until the vinegar is absorbed completely. Then put the drugs into a frying container, fry them quickly with mild fire until the drugs become dry, and then take the drugs out of the container. The amount should be 15kg vinegar per 100kg drugs.

5. Charring Radix et Rhizoma Rhei   It is to put the raw drugs into a frying container, fry them with strong fire until the drugs' outer part become black, and then take them out of the container.

6. Qingning Pill　It is processed by adding several different adjuvant materials, with complicated processing technology.

【Processing Functions】

1. Radix et Rhizoma Rhei　It has strong effect of diarrhea. It has the effect of counteracting stagnation and purging fire to remove toxin. For example, it can be used in Dachengqi Decoction.

2. Radix et Rhizoma Rhei stir – fried with wine　It can moderate the bitter flavor, cold nature and the effect of drastic purgation. It can clear away heat – toxicity in blood system in upper energizer, and strengthen the effect of promoting blood flow to remove blood stasis. For example, it can be used in Danggui Luhui Pill which is suitable for conjunctival congestion and pyogenic; Shangqing Pill which is suitable for oral ulceration; and the Xiayuxue Decoction which is suitable for stagnant blood.

3. Radix et Rhizoma Rhei steamed with wine　It can moderate the effect of purgation and has the functions of purging heat and dissipating dampness. And at the same time it strengthens the effect of promoting circulation for removing blood stasis. For example, it can be used in Dahuang Pill which is suitable for dryness of intestine and constipation; and Runchang Pill which is suitable for old people and children to loose bowel to relieve constipation.

4. Radix et Rhizoma Rhei stir – fried with vinegar　Its main functions are removing food retention and blood stasis.

5. Charring Radix et Rhizoma Rhei　It has the minimum effect of diarrhea. But it can cool the blood to remove blood stasis and has the function of hemostasis. For example, it can be used in Shihui Powder which is suitable for bleeding in stools because of retention at large intestines and hemoptysis due to pathogenic fire.

6. Qingning Pill　It has the effect of lubricant purgation and can be used for habitual constipation of old people.

【Processing Research】

There are components in Radix et Rhizoma Rhei with the effects of diarrhea, bacteriostasis, and hemostasis. After being processed, the components with diarrhea effect would be decreased, thus the side effects of diarrhea would be reduced. The studies show that the contents of binding – type anthraquinone inducing diarrhea are 2.12% in raw drugs, 2.11% in pieces of raw drugs, 1.65% in stir – fried – with – wine products, 1.04% in steamed products and 0.47% in charred products. The contents of liberation – type anthraquinone without diarrhea effect are 1.35% in raw drugs, 1.01% in pieces of raw drugs, 1.43% in stir – fried with wine products, 1.50% in steamed products and 2.60% in charred products. Meanwhile, the contents of components with the effect of hemostasis are increased, the contents of components with bacteriostasis effect remain the same.

Radix Angelicae Sinensis（Danggui）

【Source】 Radix Angelicae Sinensis is the dried root of *Angelica sinensis* (Oliv.) Diels (Fam. Umbelliferae) .

【Processing Methods】

1. Raw Radix Angelicae Sinensis　It should be purified, washed clean, moistened slightly and cut into thin slices, then exposed in the air to become dry or made dry with low heat.

2. Stir – frying Radix Angelicae Sinensis with wine　It is to put the drug slices into wine and mix them thoroughly so as to become slightly moistened. After the wine is absorbed thoroughly by the drugs, pour the drugs into a frying container, fry them quickly with mild fire until the drugs' appearances become deep yellow with a few dark spots on the surface. The amount should be 10kg wine per 100kg drugs.

3. Stir – frying Radix Angelicae Sinensis with soil　It is to put soil evenly into the frying container, which has been preheated with medium fire. Then, add drugs when the soil flows easily, fry them until the fine soil cover the pieces of drugs evenly, and the fragrant smell comes out, and then take them out. The amount should be 30kg soil per 100kg drugs.

4. Charring Radix Angelicae Sinensis　Put the drugs into a frying container and then fry them with medium fire until the drugs show a little black color on the surface and become crisp in texture.

【Processing Functions】

1. Radix Angelicae Sinensis　It has the functions of nourishing blood and lubricating intestines. For example, it can be used in Runchang Pills which could treat constipation.

2. Stir – frying Radix Angelicae Sinensis with wine　It can strengthen the effects of activating blood to promote menstruation and removing blood stasis to stop pain. It is suitable for many pain syndromes such as amenorrhea, dysmenorrheal, rheumatism, injuries from fall or fractures or contusions or strains and hemostasis swelling pain. For example, it can be used in Miraculous Decoction which could treat abscesses and swelling.

3. Stir – frying Radix Angelicae Sinensis with soil　It has the function of nourishing blood without inducing diarrhea, suitable for patients with blood deficiency and loose stool.

4. Charred Radix Angelicae Sinensis　It has the major functions of hemostasis. For example, it can be used in Yang – reviving Pill which could treat metrorrhagia and metrostaxis.

【Processing Research】

As for Radix Angelicae Sinensis, different parts have different effects owing to different components. The top part, having lower content of volatile oil than that in the tail, has the effect of hemostasis, the tail part has the effect of promoting blood flow; the body part has the effect of nourishing blood. The whole drug has the effect of regulating blood. The content of ferulic acid is the highest in raw products. If used for nourishing *qi* and blood, easing pain, and the raw products should be chosen. The content of tannin, which has the strong effect of hemostasis, is the highest in the charred products. If the purpose is to stop bleeding, the charred products would be the first choice.

Agkistrodon (Qishe)

【Source】 Agkistrodon is the dried body of *Agkistrodon acutus* (Güenther) (Fam. Viperidae) .

【Processing Methods】

1. Raw Agkistrodon Take raw Agkistrodon, remove the head and scales, and cut into sections.

2. Meat of Agkistrodon Take Agkistrodon, remove the head, moisten the drugs thoroughly with certain amount of wine, remove the scales and bones, remain the meat, and then dry it. The amount should be 20kg wine per 100kg drugs.

3. Stir – frying Agkistrodon with wine Take the sections of drugs, mix them with wine evenly, slightly moistened; after the wine is absorbed thoroughly by the drugs, pour the drugs into a frying container, fry them quickly with mild fire until the drugs' appearances become yellowish. The amount should be 20kg wine for per 100kg drugs.

【Processing Functions】

1. Agkistrodon It can only be used externally. For example, it can be used for skin itch and hyperspasmia.

2. Stir – frying Agkistrodon with wine It can moderate the bad odor of drugs, dispel wind – damp, and activate meridians to stop pain. For example, it can be used in the Baihuashe wine which could treat wind – dampness and arthralgia, and the Shexie Xuming Decoction which could treat facial distortion.

【Processing Purposes】

1. Reduce drugs' toxicity.

2. Have the synergia effect for activating meridians

3. Increase the dissolution rate of the effective components.

4. Modify the bad smell and stink.

Rhizoma Chuanxiong (Chuanxiong)

【Source】 Rhizoma Chuanxiong is the dried rhizome of *Ligusticum chuanxiong* Hort. (Fam. Umbelliferae) .

【Processing Methods】

1. Raw Rhizoma Chuanxiong Take raw drugs, remove the impurities of the drugs, clean them with water, moisten them thoroughly, cut them into thin slices, and dry them.

2. Stir – frying Rhizoma Chuanxiong with wine Take slices of Szechwan Lovage Rhizome, mix the slices with certain amount of wine evenly, moisten the slices slightly. After the wine is absorbed thoroughly by the drugs, pour the drugs into a frying container, fry them with mild fire until the slices become crisp in texture and the drugs' appearances turn into brownish color. The amount is 10kg wine for per 100kg drugs.

【Processing Functions】

1. Raw Rhizoma Chuanxiong It has the functions of promoting blood flow and *qi*, and dispelling wind to stop pain.

2. Stir – frying Rhizoma Chuanxiong with wine It can strengthen the effects of promoting blood flow and *qi* to stop pain. For example, it can be used in Chuanxiong Chatiao Powder which is suitable for headache of wind – cold type; Qianghuo Shenshi Decoction, which is suitable for headache of wind – damp type; and Chuanxiong Powder which is suitable for headache of wind – heat type.

【Processing Research】

There is a kind of alkaloid called Chuanxiongzine in Rhizoma Chuanxiong which has the sublimation nature. In order to avoid the loss of this effective component, the drugs should not be stored for a long time.

Radix Paeoniae Alba (Baishao)

【Source】 Radix Paeoniae Alba is the dried root of *Paeonia lactiflora* Pall. (Fam. Ranunculaceae) .

【Processing Methods】

1. Raw Radix Paeoniae Alba Take raw drugs, remove the impurities of the drugs, clean them with water, moisten them thoroughly, cut them into thin slices, and dry them.

2. Stir – frying Radix Paeoniae Alba with wine Take slices of drugs, mix the slices with certain amount of wine evenly, moisten the slices slightly. After the wine is absorbed thoroughly by the drugs, pour the drugs into a frying container, fry them with mild fire until the slices become crisp in texture and the drugs' appearances turn into slight yellowish color. The amount is 10kg wine for per 100kg drugs.

3. Stir – frying Radix Paeoniae Alba without adjuvant materials Put the slices of the drugs into a pan and fry with a slow fire until the drugs' surfaces turn into a slight yellowish color.

【Processing Functions】

1. Radix Paeoniae Alba It has the functions of retaining *yin* and calming livers, checking exuberant *yang* to relieve faintness. For example, it can be used in Zhengan Xifeng Decoction and Guizhi Decoction.

2. Stir – frying Radix Paeoniae Alba with wine It can minimize the sour and cold nature which would damage livers, regulate the stomach, relieve spasms and convulsions. It is suitable for chest and hypochondriac pain. For example, it can be used in Xiaoyao Powder.

3. Stir – frying Radix Paeoniae Alba without adjuvant materials It can moderate the nature of the drug, soothe liver and regulate spleen, nourish blood and astringe *yin*.

【Processing Research】

There are many effective components in this drug. To be specific, they are as follows: paeoniflorin with the effect of relieving pain, calming and spasmolysis; paeonol with the effect of anti – inflammatory and anti – thrombosis; antipyrine benzoate with the effect of spasmolysis, relieving pain and calming, and Tannin with the effect of anti – inflammatory. The research shows that there is the highest content of effective components in the peels of the drug, it should be used in clinical practice without discarding the peels so as to avoid the loss of the effective components. Meanwhile, if it is stored for a long time or in an iron container, the color would change from white to red because tannin in it is easy to be oxidized.

Section Two　　Stir – frying with Vinegar

1. Definition

Stir – frying with vinegar refers to the processing method that stir – fries purified or cut drugs with a certain amount of vinegar, and stir – fries them to a certain degree with low heat.

2. Purposes

(1) Lead the effects of drugs to the liver meridian, so as to strengthen the effects of promoting blood circulation for removing blood stasis and regulating *qi* to alleviate pain. For example, the main effect of Radix Bupleuri (*Chaihu*) stir – fried with vinegar is to relieve stagnation of *qi* of liver. The main effect of Rhizoma Corydalis (*Yanhusuo*) stir – fried with vinegar is to promote blood circulation for removing blood stasis and stop pain.

(2) Reduce drugs' toxicity and side – effects. For example, the main effect of Flos Genkwa (*Yuanhua*) stir – fried with vinegar is to remove water retention by strong diarrhea.

(3) Rectify drugs' taste and smell. For example, the main effect of Resina Olibani (*Ruxiang*) stir – fried with vinegar is to modify its bad odor.

(4) Make drugs easy to be crushed and decocted to get more effective components. For example, the texture of mineral (Pyritum – *Zirantong*) and the shellfish (Carapax et Plastrum Testudinis – *Guijia*) would be transformed from hard to crisp after being processed.

3. Technology

There are two kinds of processing technologies.

(1) Mix vinegar with drugs firstly and then fry. The operation is as follows: mix the purified or cut drugs with vinegar evenly, moisten them, put the drugs into a frying container, after the vinegar is absorbed thoroughly, fry them with mild fire to some certain degree, and take them out to become cool. The method is suitable for most dugs.

(2) Fry drugs firstly and then sprinkle vinegar on the drugs' surface. Put the purified drugs into a a frying container, then fry them to some certain degree, then sprinkle vinegar evenly on the drugs' surfaces, fry them slightly dry, take the drugs out of the container, turn them over and over again and spread out so as to become cool. This way is suitable for those drugs which are easy to stick together after being processed.

4. Amount of Adjuvant Material

The amount of adjuvant material should be 20 ~ 30kg vinegar per 100kg drugs.

5. Suitable Drugs

This processing method is suitable for those drugs with the effect of drastic hydragogue (Flos Genkwa – *Yuanhua*), drugs with the effect of soothing liver and regulating *qi* (Radix Bupleuri – *Chaihu*), blood – activating and stasis – resolving drug (Rhizoma Corydalis – *Yanhusuo*), and drugs with bad odor (Resina Olibani – *Ruxiang*).

Radix Bupleuri (Chaihu)

【Source】 Radix Bupleuri is the dried root of *Bupleurum chinense* DC. or *Bupleurum scorzonerifolium* Willd. (Fam. Umbleeiferae).

【Processing Methods】

1. Raw Radix Bupleuri　Take the raw drugs, remove the impurities and the residue stems, clean with water, moisten thoroughly, cut them into chunks and dry them.

2. Stir – frying Radix Bupleuri with vinegar　Take chunks of the drugs, mix them with a certain amount of rice vinegar evenly, moisten them thoroughly until the vinegar is absorbed completely, then pour the drugs into a frying container, fry them with mild fire until they become dry. The amount is 10kg vinegar per 100kg drugs.

3. Stir – frying Radix Bupleuri with turtle blood　Take chunks of the drugs, mix them with a certain amount of fresh turtle blood and a certain amount of cold boiled water evenly, moisten them thoroughly until the turtle blood is absorbed completely, then pour the drugs into a frying container, fry them with mild fire until they become dry. The amount is 13kg turtle blood per 100kg drugs.

【Processing Functions】

1. Raw Radix Bupleuri　It has strong nature of ascending and dispersing, so it is mostly used for dispelling pathogenic factors from body exterior to reduce heat. For example, it can be used in Xiaochaihu Decoction and Buzhong Yiqi Decoction.

2. Radix Bupleuri stir – fried with vinegar　It can moderate the nature of ascending and dispersing while strengthen the effect of dispersing stagnated hepatic *qi* to stop pain. For example, it can be used in Xiaoyao Powder.

3. Stir – frying Radix Bupleuri with turtle blood　It can strengthen the effects of supplementing *yin*, nourishing blood and restraining the nature of ascending *yang*. It is used for bone – steaming tidal fever, fever and malaria.

【Processing Research】

In the Radix Bupleuri, there is an component called saikoside which has the functions of calming, relieving pain, cough and heat. After being processed with vinegar and under the condition of acidity, saikoside would be hydrolyzed into saikogenin whose main effects are relieving pain, cough and anti – inflammatory. Meanwhile, alph – Chondrillasterol, the main ingredient of relieving fever in this drug, would also be hydrolyzed into ester component under the condition of acidity, leading the effect of relieving fever disappear. So the main effect of stir – frying Radix Bupleuri with vinegar is to disperse stagnated hepatic *qi* to stop pain rather than reduce fever.

Rhizoma Corydalis (Yanhusuo)

【Source】 Rhizoma Corydalis is the dried tuber of *Corydalis yanhusuo* W. T. Wang (Fam. Papaveraceae).

【Processing Methods】

1. Raw Rhizoma Corydalis Take the raw drugs, clean with water, moisten thoroughly, cut them into chunks.

2. Stir – frying Rhizome Corydalis with vinegar Take purified Rhizome Corydalis, mix them with a certain amount of rice vinegar evenly, moisten them thoroughly until the vinegar is absorbed completely, then pour the drugs into a frying container, fry them with mild fire until they become dry, take them out to make them cool. The amount is 20kg vinegar per 100kg drugs.

3. Boiling Rhizome Corydalis with vinegar Take purified Rhizome Corydalis, mix them with a certain amount of rice vinegar and clean water evenly (the water just covers the drugs), then pour the drugs into a boiling container, heating them with mild fire thoroughly, take them out, cut them into chunks, and exposed in the air so as to become dry. Make them cool down. The amount is 20kg vinegar per 100kg drugs.

4. Steaming Rhizome Corydalis with vinegar Take purified Rhizome Corydalis, mix them with a certain amount of rice vinegar evenly, steaming until the vinegar is absorbed completely, take them out, cut them into chunks, and exposed drugs in the air so as to make them dry. The amount is 20kg vinegar per 100kg drugs.

【Processing Functions】

1. Raw Rhizoma Corydalis Rarely applied in clinical practice.

2. Stir – frying Rhizoma Corydalis with vinegar It can strengthen the effects of promoting blood circulation, activating *qi*, and stopping pain. For example, it can be used in Wujin Pills and Yanhu Zhitong Pills.

【Processing Research】

After being processed with vinegar, the effect of relieving pain would be strengthened. The first reason is that the synergistic action occurs by the drugs being processed with vinegar (the effect can be conducted to liver meridian). The second reason is that the pain – relieving component free tetrahydropalmatine is transfered to alkaloid salt and easy to be decocted after the drug being processed with vinegar.

The study shows that the contents of total alkaloid are 25.06% in raw ingredients, 49.33% in the products stir – fried with vinegar, and 22.66% in the products stir – fried with wine.

Furthermore, the dissolution rates of effective components are also influenced by different ratios and different kinds of the acids. For example, the decoction ratios by using tartaric acid are

68. 02% and 64. 66% by using citric acid, which are all higher than that by using normal vinegar.

Olibanum (Ruxiang)

【Source】Olibanum is the dried resin of *Boswellia carterii* Birdw or *Boswellia bhawdajiana* Birdw. (Fam. Burseraceae) .

【Processing Methods】

1. Raw Olibanum   Take the raw drugs, remove the impurities, and break the large – size ones into smaller ones.

2. Stir – frying Olibanum with vinegar   Take purified drugs, pour the drugs into a frying container, fry them with mild fire until the drugs smoke and become slightly melted. Then, sprinkle a certain amount of rice vinegar evenly on the drugs' surface, fry with mild fire until the drugs show a greasy luster, then take them out quickly and spread them out to air so as to become dry. The amount is 10kg vinegar per 100kg drugs.

3. Stir – frying Olibanum without adjuvant materials   Take purified drugs, pour the drugs into a frying container, fry them with mild fire until the drugs smoke and show a greasy luster, then take them out quickly and spread them out to air so as to become dry.

【Processing Functions】

1. Raw Olibanum   It has strong irritation to stomachs and is easy to cause vomiting, therefore it is only used externally. For example, it can be used in making Jiushengren Powder which are suitable for fracture.

2. Stir – frying Olibanum with vinegar   Its taste and smell has been modified. The processing has synergistic action of strengthening the effects of promoting blood circulation to arrest pain, astringing and promoting tissue regeneration.

3. Stir – frying Olibanum without adjuvant materials   It can reduce the drugs' irritation and make them easy to be crushed.

【Processing Research】

There are resin, gum and volatile oil in this drug. The content of the resin is 60% ~70% and that of the gum is 27 % ~35%. The volatile oil is the simulating component. After being processed with vinegar, most of the volatile oil is eliminated, leading the irritation to reduce.

Flos Genkwa (Yuanhua)

【Source】Flos Genkwa is the dried flower bud of *Daphne genkwa* Sieb. et Zucc. (Fam. Thymelaeaceae) .

【Processing Methods】

1. Raw Flos Genkwa   Take the raw drugs, remove the impurities, stems and leaves.

2. Stir – frying Flos Genkwa with vinegar   Take purified drugs, mix them with a certain amount of rice vinegar evenly, moisten them thoroughly until the vinegar is absorbed completely, then pour the drugs into a frying container, fry them with mild fire until they become slightly

dry. The amount is 30kg vinegar per 100kg drugs.

3. Boiling Flos Genkwa with vinegar　Take purified drugs, put them into a boiling container, mix them with a certain amount of rice vinegar evenly, boil them until the vinegar is absorbed completely by the drugs. The amount is 30 ~ 40kg vinegar and 30kg water per 100kg drugs.

【Processing Functions】

1. Raw Flos Genkwa　It is toxical, having effects of drastic hydragogue, only used externally. For example, it can be used in Yuanhua Powder which is suitable for toothache.

2. Stir – frying Flos Genkwa with vinegar　It can reduce the toxicity, moderate the effect of removing water retention by strong diarrhea. For example, it can be used in Zhouche pills and Shizao Decoction.

【Processing Purposes】

1. Reduce the toxicity.

2. Moderate the effect of diarrhea and the syndrome of stomachache.

【Processing Research】

After being processed with vinegar, under the condition of acidity, flavonoid glycoside in this drug would be hydrolyzed into genkwanin, whose main effect is to eliminate phlegm. Meanwhile, the unsaturated volatile oil causing irritation would also be changed. The study shows that acute toxicity LD_{50} of alcohol extract of raw products and stir – fried with vinegar products are 1.0% and 7.07% respectively. Water extract of raw products and stir – fried with vinegar products are 8.3% and 17.78% respectively. The results indicate that after being processed, the toxicity of Flos Genkwa would undoubtedly be reduced.

Section Three　Stir – frying with Salt Water

1. Definition

Stir – frying with salt solution refers to the processing method that mixes a certain amount of salt solution with purified or cut drugs and stir – fries them with mild fire.

2. Purposes

(1) The processing method helps to conduct the effects of drugs to the kidney meridian. For example, the main effects of the raw drugs of Cortex Eucommiae (*Duzhong*) are to replenish liver and kidney, to strengthen muscle and bone, and to prevent abortion. After being processed with salt solution, the effects of the drug would be conducted to kidney meridian and would be strengthened.

(2) Stir – frying with salt solution could enhance drugs' effects. For example, the main effects of raw products of Cortex Phellodendri Chinensis (*Huangbo*) are to purge pathogenic fire, detoxicate and clear heat and dry dampness. After being stir – fried with salt solution, the bitter

taste and dryness of the raw drug would be moderated. The effects could be conducted to kidney meridian so as to purge away pathogenic fire in kidney.

(3) Moderate drugs' nature. For example, the pungent and dry nature of Fructus Psoraleae (*Buguzhi*) would be moderated after being processed with salt solution.

3. Technology

There are two kinds of processing technologies.

(1) The first way is to mix drugs with salt solution first then fry. It is suitable for most drugs.

Mix the drugs with salt solution evenly, moisten them thoroughly, put them into a frying container, then fry them with mild fire until the salt solution is absorbed completely, then take the drugs out of the container so as to make them cool.

(2) The second way is to fry drugs first and then sprinkle salt solution on drugs' surface. It is suitable for those drugs with phlegmatic temperament (such as Semen Plantaginis – *Cheqianzi*).

Put drugs into a frying container and fry with mild fire to a certain degree, then sprinkle salt solution evenly on the drugs' surface and fry them until they become. Finally, take the drugs out and make them become cool.

4. Amount of Adjuvant Material

The amount of adjuvant material should be 2kg salt with 8kg ~ 10kg water per 100kg drugs.

5. Suitable Drugs

This method is suitable for those drugs with the effects of invigorating kidney and astringing fluid, treating hernia, promoting diuresis and purging the kidney heat.

Semen Plantaginis (Cheqianzi)

【Source】Semen Plantaginis is the dried ripe seed of *Plantago asiatica* L. or *Plantago depressa* Willd. (Fam. Plantaginaceae).

【Processing Methods】

1. Raw Semen Plantaginis   Take the raw drugs, remove the impurities.

2. Stir – frying Semen Plantaginis with salt solution   Put purified raw plantain seed into a frying container, stir – fry them with mild fire till the seeds begin to crack slightly, then sprinkle salt water evenly on the drugs' surface and fry them until the drugs become dry. Finally, take out the drugs and make them cool.

3. Stir – frying Semen Plantaginis without adjuvant materials   Put the purified raw drugs into a pan and stir – fry with a mild fire till the seeds begin to crack slightly and with a nice smell, take out the drugs and make them become cool.

【Processing Functions】

1. Raw Semen Plantaginis   It is sweet in flavor, cold in nature, has the functions of clearing away heat and treating stranguria. For example, it can be used in Cheqianzi Powder which is suitable for stranguria, conjunctival congestion and swelling.

2. Semen Plantaginis stir – fried with salt solution　It can replenish liver and kidney, improve vision, and alleviate water retention. For example, it can be used in Zhujing Pills for replenishing liver and kidney, and improving vision.

3. Stir – frying Semen Plantaginis without adjuvant materials　It can moderate the cold nature of the raw drugs and remove water – damp without damaging *qi* of spleens. For example, it can be used in Siling Powder for treating accumulation of dampness and diarrhea due to *qi* deficiency of spleens.

【Processing Research】

After being processed with salt solution, the content of the flavonoid would be changed and the decoction ratio of effective components would be increased. The study shows that the decoction ratios of effective components are 71.32% in the raw drugs, 81% in stir – fried with salt solution products, and 84.70% in stir – fried without adjuvant materials products.

Contex Phellodendri Chinensis (Huangbo)

【Source】Contex Phellodendri is Chinensis the dried bark of *Phellodendron chinensis* Schneid. (Fam. Rutaceae).

【Processing Methods】

1. Raw Contex Phellodendri Chinensis　Take the raw drugs, remove the impurities, discard its cork layers, clean them with water, moisten thoroughly, cut them into filaments or dominoes pieces, and dry them.

2. Stir – frying Contex Phellodendri Chinensis with salt solution　Mix the filaments or dominoes pieces of the drugs with salt solution evenly, moisten them slightly, after the salt solution is absorbed thoroughly, put the drugs into a frying container, fry them with mild fire until the drugs' outer parts become deep yellowish with focal spots. In this processing method, 100kg drugs should be stir – fried with 2kg salt.

3. Stir – frying Contex Phellodendri Chinensis with wine　Mix the filaments or dominoes pieces of the drugs with yellowish wine evenly, moisten them slightly, after the yellowish wine is absorbed thoroughly, put the drugs into a frying container, fry them with mild fire until the drugs' outer parts become slightly yellowish, and nice smell of wine flows. In this processing method, 100kg drugs should be stir – fried with 10kg wine.

4. Charring Contex Phellodendri Chinensis　Put the filaments of the drugs into a frying container, fry them with strong fire until the drugs become burned – black outside and puce inside.

【Processing Functions】

1. Raw Contex Phellodendri Chinensis　It has the functions of purging fire and removing toxin, and eliminating heat and dampness. For example, it can be used in Baitouweng Decoction for treating damp – heat dysentery, Zhizi Baipi Decoction for treating jaundice.

2. Stir – frying Contex Phellodendri Chinensis with salt solution　It can moderate the bitter and dry nature of the raw drugs , concentrate the effects on the kidney meridian, purge away ministerial fire. For example, it can be used in Dabuyin Pills for treating *yin* deficiency with bone – steaming, night sweat and seminal emission.

3. Stir – frying Contex Phellodendri Chinensis with wine
It can elevate the effects, moderate the bitter and cold nature of the raw drugs, and expel dampness heat in upper energizer. For example, it can be used in Shangqing Pills for treating conjunctival congestion and swollen sore throat.

4. Charred Contex Phellodendri Chinensis
It is bitter in flavor and astringent in nature, having the effect of hemostasis by clearing away heat. It can be used for hematuria, metrorrhagia and metrostaxis.

Except for the four processing methods mentioned above, there is still another processing method, for example, stir – frying Contex Phellodendri Chinensis with honey, which could be used to treat oral ulceration.

【Processing Research】

The content of berberine would be influenced by water processing. In order to avoid the loss of the effective ingredients, it should be washed quickly during the purifying and cutting process, and cut them into pieces timely. Furthermore, the content of berberine would also change after being stir – fried. The study shows that the contents of berberine are 100% , 96% , 87% and 16% in the raw drugs, the products stir – fried with wine, the products stir – fried with salt solution and the charred products respectively.

Cortex Eucommiae (Duzhong)

【Source】 Cortex Eucommiaceae is the dried stem bark of *Eucommia ulmoides* Oliv. (Fam. Eucom – miaceae) .

【Processing Methods】

1. Raw Cortex Eucommiae
It should be removed its cork layers, washed, moistened thoroughly and cut into filaments or clumps.

2. Stir – frying Cortex Eucommiae with salt solution
Mix the filaments of the drugs and salt solution evenly, moisten them slightly, after the salt solution is absorbed thoroughly, put the drugs into a frying container and fry them with medium fire until the drugs' outer parts show a coke brown color or a burned black color and become easy to be broken, then, take them out to make them become cool. In this processing method, 100kg drugs should be stir – fried with 2kg salt.

【Processing Functions】

1. Raw Cortex Eucommiae
It has the functions of replenishing liver and kidney, strengthening muscle & bone, and preventing abortion.

2. Cortex Eucommiae stir – fried with salt water
It could be concentrated on the kidney meridian, strengthening the effects mentioned above. For example, it can be used in Qinge Pills for treating lumbago due to kidney deficiency; Duzhong Jiangya Pill for treating hypertension.

【Processing Research】

The study shows that the decoction ratios of effective components are 10. 37% in raw drugs and 18. 44% in stir – fried with salt solution products. Pharmacological tests show that the drugs stir – fried with salt solution have a stronger pharmacologic action of depressurization than that of raw drugs.

Section Four　Stir – frying with Ginger Juice

1. Definition

Stir – frying with ginger juice refers to the processing method that to mix a certain amount of ginger juice with the purified or cut drugs and stir – fry them with mild fire to some degree.

2. The Purposes

(1) Moderate drugs' nature. For example, the nature of raw products of Rhizoma Coptidis (*Huanglian*) is bitter and cold, after being processed with ginger juice, the nature could be moderated.

(2) Strengthen the drugs' effect of regulating stomachs to stop vomiting. For example, after being processed with ginger juice, Rhizoma Coptidis (*Huanglian*) could stop vomiting, Fructus Amomi (*Sharen*) could warm stomachs to stop vomiting, and Caulis Bambusae in Taenia (*Zhu-ru*) could calm adverse – rising energy to stop vomiting.

(3) Reduce drugs' irritation. For example, the main effect of the raw products of Cortex Magnoliae Officinalis (*Houpo*) is likely to stimulate throats. After being stir – fried with ginger juice, the irritation could be reduced; the effects of warming middle – energizer, resolving dampness and relieving stagnation of *qi* could be strengthened. The raw products of Rhizoma Pinelliae (*Banxia*) has irritation and astringency, after being stir – fried with ginger juice, the irritation could be reduced, the effect of calming adverse – rising energy to stop vomiting would be strengthened.

3. Technology

There are two kinds of processing technologies.

(1) The first way is to mix ginger juice with drugs first and then to fry. Ginger juice could be got by grinding fresh ginger or decocting Zingiberis rhizome.

To be specific, it is to put drugs and ginger juice together, mix them thoroughly and moisten them completely, make the ginger juice penetrate gradually into the inner parts of the drugs. Put the drugs into a frying container and fry them with mild fire to some certain degree, and finally take the drugs out and make them become cool.

(2) The second way is to boil drugs with ginger juice together. Firstly, boil the fresh ginger

and some water together to get ginger juice. Then, add the drugs into the juice and continue to boil for two hours. When the ginger juice is almost absorbed by the drugs, take out the drugs, dry them and cut them into slices.

4. Amount of Adjuvant Material

The amount of adjuvant materials needed in the processing should be 10kg fresh ginger or 10/3kg Zingiberis Rhizoma per 100kg drugs.

5. Suitable Drugs

This processing method is suitable for those drugs with the effects of stopping coughing and eliminating phlegm and checking adverse rise of *qi* to stop vomiting.

Cortex Magnoliae Officinalis (Houpo)

【Source】 Cortex Magnoliae Officinalis is the dried stem bark, root bark or branch bark of *Magnolia officinalis* Rehd. et Wils. or *Magnolia officinalis* Rehd. et Wils. var. *biloba* Rehd. et Wils. (Fam. Magnoliaceae).

【Processing Methods】

1. Raw Cortex Magnoliae officinalis　Take the raw drugs, discard their cork layers, clean them with water, moisten thoroughly, cut them into filaments, and dry them.

2. Stir－frying Cortex Magnoliae officinalis with ginger juice　Mix the filaments of the drugs with ginger juice evenly, moisten them thoroughly, after the ginger juice is thoroughly absorbed, put the drugs into a frying container, fry them with mild fire to become dry.

3. Boiling Cortex Magnoliae officinalis with ginger juice　Take ginger slices and decoct them, band drugs whose cork layers have been discarded into bundles, and then put into the ginger decoction, showering the drugs with the ginger juice over and over again; boiling with mild fire until the ginger juice is absorbed completely. Finally, take the drugs out, cut into filaments and make them become dry. In the processing method, 100kg raw drugs should be processed with 10kg fresh ginger or 10/3kg Zingiberis Rhizoma per 100kg drugs.

【Processing Functions】

1. Raw Cortex Magnoliae officinalis　It has the effects of depriving evil wetness and dispersing phlegm, descending *qi* and eliminating stagnation. For the raw product has drastic action and irritation to throats, it is seldom advised to take orally.

2. Cortex Magnoliae officinalis processed with ginger juice　It can reduce the irritation to throats and strengthen the effects of warming the middle energizer and regulating the function of the stomachs. For example, it can be used in Pingwei Powder treating in splenic－gastric wet detention.

【Main Purposes】

1. Reduce irritation of the drug.

2. Strengthen the synergistic action and efficacy.

【Processing Research】

The purpose of discarding the cork layers is to enhance the relative contents of effective components. The main effects of magnolol or honokiol in this drug are antibiosis, calming and anti – gastric ulcer. The main effects of volatile oil in it are calming, perspiring, eliminating phlegm and relieving asthma. After being processed with ginger juice, the contents of components mentioned above are all increased or changed.

Caulis Bambusae in Taeniam (Zhuru)

【Source】 Caulis Bambusae in Taeniamis the dried middle shavings of stem of *Bambusa tuldoides* Munro, *Sinocalamus beecheyanus* (Munro) McClure var. *pubescens* P. F. Li or *Phyllostachys nigra* (Lodd.) Munro var. *henonis* (Mitf.) Stapf ex Rendle (Fam. Gramineae).

【Processing Methods】

1. Raw Caulis Bambusae in Taeniam
Take the raw drugs, remove the foreign materials and sclerodermite, cut them into sections or malaxate them into small balls.

2. Stir – frying Caulis Bambusae in Taeniam with ginger juice
Mix ginger juice with sections or balls of Caulis Bambusae in Teaniam evenly, moisten them slightly, after the ginger juice is absorbed thoroughly, put the drugs into a frying container, fry them with mild fire, iron the drugs until they show a yellowish color, then, take the drugs out and make them become cool. In this processing method, 10kg fresh ginger is needed to be processed per 100kg drugs.

【Processing Functions】

1. Raw Caulis Bambusae in Taeniam
It has the functions of cleaning and resolving heat phlegm, it can be used to treat hemoptysis due to lung heat.

2. Caulis Bambusae in Taeniam stir – fried with ginger juice
It can strengthen the effect of checking adverse rise of *qi* to stop vomiting. For example, it can be used in Jupi Zhuru Decoction for treating the syndromes of stomach deficiency with heat and vomiting.

Section Five   Stir – frying with Honey

1. Definition

Stir – frying with honey refers to the processing method that mixes refined honey into purified or cut drugs and stir – fries them with mild fire to some degree. In this method, the honey should be refined by heating before using in processing.

2. Purposes

(1) Honey has synergistic action and could enhance drugs' effectiveness. For example, the main effect of the raw product of Radix Stemonae (*Baibu*) is to stop coughing and eliminate phlegm. After they are stir – fried with honey, the effect of moistening lung and stopping cough

would be strengthened. The main effect of raw product of Radix Astragali (*Huangqi*) is to tonify *qi* and strengthen the exterior. After they are stir – fried with honey, the synergistic action of honey could strengthen the effect of tonifying the middle energizer and invigorating *qi*.

(2) Honey helps to moderate drugs' nature. For example, the raw product of Fructus Aristolochiae (*Madouling*) is bitter in flavor and cold in nature, and has the effects of clearing heat of lung and depressing *qi* and relieving cough and asthma. After it is stir – fried with honey, the nature could be moderated, and the effect of moistening lung and stopping coughing could be strengthened. The raw product of Herba Ephedrae (*Mahuang*) has the functions of inducing sweating and dispelling exogenous evils. After they are stir – fried with honey, the pungent dispersing and perspiration effect could be moderated. The main effect is to disperse lung *qi* to stop asthma.

(3) Honey helps to modify the drugs' taste and eliminate the side effects. For example, the raw product of Fructus Aristolochiae (*Madouling*) is easy to cause nausea and vomiting, after they are stir – fried with honey, the bad taste could be moderated and the side effect of vomiting could be eliminated.

3. Technology

There are two kinds of processing technologies.

(1) The first way suitable for the drugs with crisp texture is to mix honey with drugs first and then fry.

Dilute some refined honey with a certain amount of boiled water, then put drugs into the honey, mix thoroughly and moisten thoroughly, and make the honey penetrate into the inner part of the drugs; put the drugs into a preheating pan and fry them with mild fire until the drugs show a deep color and with no sticking. Finally, take the drugs out of the pan and spread them to make them become cool.

(2) The second way suitable for those drugs of dense texture is to fry drugs first and then sprinkle honey on drugs' surface.

Put drugs into a preheating pan and fry with mild fire, when the drugs become deep in color, pour some refined honey evenly on the drugs' surface and fry quickly, mix them thoroughly; when there is no sticking, take the drugs out of the pan and spread them to make them become cool.

4. Amount of Adjuvant Material

The amount of adjuvant material needed in the processing is normally 25kg honey per 100kg drugs.

5. Suitable Drugs

This method is suitable for the drugs with effects of relieving cough and asthma and invigorating middle energizer and tonifying *qi*.

6. Notice

(1) The refined honey should be diluted with boiled water to make it not so viscous.

（2）The drugs and the refined honey should be mixed fully and moistened thoroughly. This is to make sure that the honey could penetrate into the inner parts of the drugs.

（3）During the process, the power should be mild so as not to parch the drugs.

（4）The drugs processed with honey should be stored and placed at cool places, avoiding sun light and with the container closed tightly.

Radix Glycyrrhizae (Gancao)

【Source】 Radix Glycyrrhizae is the dried root and rhizome of *Glycyrrhiza uralensis* Fisch. , *Glycyrrhiza inflate* Bat. Or *Glycyrrhiza glabra* L. (Fam. Leguminosae) .

【Processing Methods】

1. Raw Radix Glycyrrhizae Take the raw drugs, remove the impurities, clean them with water, moisten thoroughly, cut them into junks, and dry them in the sun.

2. Stir – frying Raw Radix Glycyrrhizae with honey Take some refined honey, dilute it with boiled water, shower the honey into the purified slices of the drugs and mix them thoroughly, moisten the drugs. Put the drugs into a frying container and fry them with mild fire till the drugs show a deep yellow color and with no sticking, take them out and make them become cool. In the processing, it needs 25kg honey per 100kg drugs.

【Processing Functions】

1. Raw Radix Glycyrrhizae It is good at purging fire and detoxification, preventing phlegm and stopping coughing. For example, it can be used in Yinhua Gancao Decoction for treating diseases of swelling and ulcer; Shashen Maidong Decoction for treating coughing due to fever and phlegm, and Jiegeng Decoction for treating swollen sore throat.

2. Radix Glycyrrhizae stir – fried with honey It can invigorate spleens, benefit middle energizer, relieve spasm, and stop pain. For example, it can be used in Sijunzi Decoction and Zhigancao Decoction.

【Processing Research】

Radix Glycyrrhizae has the effect of protecting mucosa to relieve cough and good effect of detoxification. The reasons of detoxification are as follows: ①It has the same effect as that of epinephrine; ②It can help to enhance the detoxification of the liver; ③It can help to absorb the toxic ingredients; ④The derivation of Glycyrrhizic acid is Glucuronic acid, which could be combined with toxic components.

The study shows that when Radix Glycyrrhizae is made softened before cut, the wastage ratios of water extract are 49. 89% by soaking with water for 48 hours, and 7. 22% by moistening with water for 48 hours. The wastage ratios of glycyrrhizic acid in the two products are 48. 40% and 4. 99% respectively. The thickness of the piece also influences the extract ratio of glycyrrhizic acid. For example, the extract ratios are 99. 91% in the pieces of 2 ~ 3mm and 85. 22% in the pieces of 5 ~ 6mm.

Herba Ephedra (Mahuang)

【Source】 Herba Ephedra is the dried herbaceous stem of *Ephedra sinica* Stapf, Ephedra *in-*

termedia Schrenk et C. A. Mey. or *Ephedra equisetina* Bge. (Fam. Ephedraceae) .

【Processing Methods】

1. Raw Herba Ephedra
Take the raw drugs, remove xylon stem, nub and impurities, moisten slightly, cut them into sections, and dry them.

2. Stir－frying Herba Ephedra with honey
Dilute some refined honey with boiled water, shower the honey into the purified sections of the drugs and mix them thoroughly until they are moistened the drugs. Put the drugs into a pot and fry with a mild fire till the drugs become not sticking, take them out and make them become cool. This processing needs 20kg honey per 100kg drugs.

3. Herba Ephedra velvet
Grind drugs to velvet and screen out fine powders.

4. Stir－frying Herba Ephedra with honey of velvet
Dilute some refined honey with boiled water, shower the honey into the velvets of the drugs and mix them evenly until they are moistened thoroughly, put the drugs into a frying container, fry them with mild fire till the drugs show a deep yellow color without sticking, take them out and make them become cool, 25kg honey per 100kg drugs.

【Processing Functions】

1. Raw Herba Ephedra
It has the effects of inducing sweating and dispelling exogenous evils, dispersing lung *qi* & relieving asthma, and inducing diuresis to alleviate edema. For example, it can be used in Mahuang Decoction for treating wind－coldness due to exterior infection and the syndromes of exterior excess coldness without sweat, Yuebi Decoction for treating the syndromes of edema, aversion to wind and face edema caused by wind－evil.

2. Herba Ephedra stir－fried with honey
It can moderate the effect of inducing sweating but strengthen the function of dispersing lung *qi* to relieve asthma and stop coughing. For example, it can be used in Sanniu Decoction for treating less exterior syndrome but more cough.

3. Herba Ephedra velvet
It can greatly moderate the effect of inducing sweating and dispelling exogenous evils, has the function of inducing diuresis alleviate edema. It can be used for wind cold of the old people and children.

4. Herba Ephedra velvet stir－fried with honey
Relieve cough and asthma, used for uncured cough and dyspnea without exterior syndromes.

【Processing Research】

The content of alkaloid in this drug changes little and volatile oil decreases after being processed. The roots and stalks have different uses, they should be used differently in clinical practice.

Section Six　Stir－frying with Oil

1. Definition

Stir－frying with oil refers to the processing method that co－heats purified or cut drugs with a certain amount of oil.

2. Purposes

(1) Strengthen drugs' effect of warming kidney to invigorate *yang*.

(2) Make drugs easy to be crushed, facilitate preparation and taking.

3. Technology

There are three kinds of processing technologies.

(1) Stir – frying with oil. Mix drugs with oil evenly, put them into a frying container, fry them quickly with mild fire until the oil is absorbed thoroughly by the drugs. 20kg oil per 100kg drugs.

(2) Frying drugs in oil. Heat oil in a pot until it boils, then pour the drugs in and fry them deeply with mild fire until the drugs become crisp. 25kg oil per 100kg drugs.

(3) Baking drugs with oil. Cut drugs into clumps, bake them on fire, coat the drugs with oil and bake until the oil penetrates into the inner parts of the drugs, repeat the coating and baking procedure until the drugs become crisp.

Herba Epimedii (Yinyanghuo)

【Source】 Herba Epimedii is the dried foliage of *Epimedium brevicornu* Maxim. , *Epimedium sagittatum* (Sieb. et Zucc.) Maxim. , *Epimedium pubescens* Maxim. or *Epimedium koreanum* Nakai (Fam. Berberidaceae) .

【Processing Methods】

1. Raw Herba Epimedii Take the raw drugs, remove the impurities, moisten them slightly, cut them into filaments, and dry them.

2. Stir – frying Herba Epimedii with oil Melt some sheep's oil first and then put the drug filaments into it, fry the drugs with mild fire until the oil is absorbed thoroughly until the drugs become yellowish and slightly shiny. Finally, take the drugs out of the pot. This processing needs 20kg refined oil per 100kg drugs.

【Processing Functions】

1. Raw Herba Epimedii It can expel wind – evil and remove wetness and strengthen muscles and bone. For example, it can be used in Yinyanghuo Powder and Yinyanghuo Pills.

2. Herba Epimedii stir – fried with oil It can tonify kidney and invigorate *yang*. For example, it can be used in Sanshen Pills which are used for treating feebleness of kidney – *qi*.

Gecko (Gejie)

【Source】 Gecko is the dried body of *Gekko gecko* Linnaeus (Fam. Gekkonidae) .

【Processing Methods】

1. Raw Gecko Take the raw drugs, remove the bamboo pieces and then clean them with water; remove heads, feet, claws and scales, cut them into clumps and make them become dry.

2. Stir – frying Gecko with wine　　Mix clumps of Gecko with wine evenly until they are moistened, after the wine is absorbed thoroughly, put the drugs into a frying container, fry them with mild fire until the drugs become dry. This processing needs 20kg wine per 100kg drugs.

3. Baking Gecko with overlaying oil　　Bake clumps of Gecko on fire with overlaying teel oil until the drugs show a yellow color and a crisp texture, then cut the clumps into smaller ones.

【Processing Functions】

1. Raw Gecko　　It has the functions of invigorating lung and kidney, reliving asthma and tonifying *yang* to profit essence.

2. Gecko stir – fried with wine　　It can strengthen the effect of invigorating kidney and tonifying *yang*.

3. Gecko baked with overlaying oil　　It has the same effects as those of raw Gecko. Furthermore, this processing method makes them crisp and easier to be crushed, moderate the bad odor.

第九章 炙 法

1. 定义

将净选或切制后的药物，加入一定量的液体辅料拌炒，使辅料逐渐渗入药物组织内部的炮制方法。

2. 种类

炙法根据所用辅料不同，可分为酒炙、醋炙、盐炙、姜炙、蜜炙、油炙等法。

3. 炙法与加固体辅料炒法的区别

加固体辅料炒法与加液体辅料炒法在一些方面有所区别，如下表：

	液体辅料	固体辅料
温 度	文火	中火或武火
时 间	长	短
过 程	辅料渗透入药物	辅料不渗透入药物
性 质	辅料使大多数药物的理化性质发生改变	辅料主要作为热传导介质，增强药效，使药物表面颜色加深
操作方法	先对药物进行炒制，然后加入辅料；或者先将药物与辅料拌匀，然后进行炒制	先对辅料进行加热，然后加入药物

4. 分类

根据所加辅料可分为如下几类：酒炙法，例如大黄；醋炙法，例如甘遂；盐炙法，例如黄柏；姜炙法，例如厚朴；蜜炙法，例如麻黄；油炙法，例如三七。

第一节 酒 炙 法

1. 定义

将净选或切制后的药物，加入一定量酒，用文火拌炒至一定程度的方法。

2. 目的

（1）改变药性。例如，龙胆主要功效为清热泻火燥湿，但是经过酒炙之后，则用于肝胆实火所致的头胀头痛以及目赤肿痛。

（2）协同作用。经过炮制之后，药物活血通络的作用得到增强，如当归。

（3）缓和药性。经过炮制之后，药物的寒凉之性得以缓和，如黄连。

（4）提高药物有效成分的溶出率。药物经过炮制，其有效成分溶出率增大，增强了疗效，如黄芩。

（5）矫臭去腥。一些具有腥气的动物类药物，经过炮制后可除去或减弱腥臭气，如乌梢蛇。

（6）降低药物的毒副作用，并使其质地酥脆易于粉碎，如蟾酥。

3. 工艺

酒炙法有两种工艺。

（1）先拌酒后炒药。适用于大多数药物，特别适用于质地较坚实的根茎类药物。

将净制或切制后的药物与一定量的酒拌匀，稍闷润，待酒被吸尽后，置炒制容器内，用文火炒干。

（2）先炒药后加酒。适用于质地疏松的药物，如五灵脂。

先将净制或切制后的药物，置炒制容器内，加热至一定程度，再喷洒一定量的酒炒干。

4. 用量

一般每100kg药物，用黄酒10～20kg。

5. 适用药物

（1）性质苦寒的药物，如大黄。

（2）活血祛瘀的药物，如当归。

（3）祛风通络的药物，如威灵仙。

黄　　连

【来源】本品为毛茛科植物黄连、三角叶黄连或云连的干燥根茎。

【炮制方法】

1. **黄连**　取原药材，除去杂质，抢水洗净，润透，切薄片。

2. **酒黄连**　取黄连片，加入定量黄酒拌匀，稍闷润，待酒被吸尽后，置炒制容器内，用文火加热，炒干。每100kg黄连片，用黄酒12.5kg。

3. **萸黄连**　取吴茱萸加适量水煎煮，取汁去渣，煎液与黄连片拌匀，稍闷润，待药液被吸尽后，置炒制容器内，用文火加热，炒干。每100kg黄连片，用吴茱萸10kg。

4. **姜黄连**　取黄连片，用姜汁拌匀，稍闷润，待姜汁被吸尽后，置炒制容器内，用文火加热炒干。每100kg黄连片，用生姜10kg。

【炮制作用】

1. **生黄连** 苦寒性强，长于清热燥湿，清心火，如用于治疗热毒雍盛的黄连解毒汤，及治疗血热妄行的泻心汤。

2. **酒黄连** 增强药效并缓和苦寒之性，上清上焦火热，用于目赤肿痛，口舌生疮。

3. **萸黄连** 苦、寒之性缓和，寒而不滞，治肝郁化火，清气分湿热，散肝胆郁火，如用于治疗湿热泻泄香连丸。

4. **姜黄连** 清胃止呕，用于治疗胃热呕吐的半夏泻心汤。

【炮制研究】

黄连在进行炮制之前应抢水洗净，以避免有效成分的流失。黄连经过炮制虽缓和了其寒凉之性，但仍苦寒败胃，因此不宜过量或者长期服用。此外，药物有效成分的溶出率随片型的不同而有所区别，其有效成分在黄连片、条、粗粉和细粉中的溶出率分别为26.34%、47.50%、58.17% 和72.43%。

大　黄

【来源】本品为蓼科植物掌叶大黄、唐古特大黄或药用大黄的干燥根及根茎。

【炮制方法】

1. **大黄** 取原药材，除去杂质，大小分开，洗净，捞出，淋润至软后，切厚片或小方块，晾干或低温干燥。

2. **酒大黄** 取大黄片或块，用黄酒喷淋拌匀，稍闷润，待酒被吸尽后，置炒制容器内，用文火炒干。每100kg 大黄片或块，用黄酒10kg。

3. **熟大黄** 取大黄片或块，用黄酒拌匀，闷至酒被吸尽，隔水炖至大黄内外均呈黑色时，取出。每100kg 大黄片或块，用黄酒30kg。

4. **醋大黄** 取大黄片或块，用米醋拌匀，稍闷润，待醋被吸尽后，置炒制容器内，用文火加热，炒干，取出。每100kg 大黄片或块，用米醋15kg。

5. **大黄炭** 取大黄片或块，置炒制容器内，用武火加热，炒至外表呈黑色时，取出。

6. **清宁片** 采用多种辅料，经过复杂炮制工艺加工而成。

【炮制作用】

1. **大黄** 泻下作用峻烈，具有攻积导滞、泻火解毒的功能，如用于大承气汤。

2. **酒大黄** 苦寒泻下作用稍缓，并借酒升提之性，善清上焦血分热毒。如用于治疗结膜充血与化脓的当归芦荟片；用于治疗口腔溃疡的上清片；治疗瘀血内停的下瘀血汤。

3. **熟大黄** 泻下作用缓和，清热除湿，并能增强活血祛瘀之功。如治疗燥结便秘的大黄丸；用于老人及小儿润肠通便的润肠丸。

4. **醋大黄** 以消积化瘀为主。

5. **大黄炭** 泻下作用极微，并有凉血化瘀止血作用。如治大肠有积滞的大便出血及热邪伤络，血不循经之呕血、咯血的十灰散。

6. **清宁片** 润肠通便。用于治疗年老者习惯性便秘。

【炮制研究】

大黄中含有具有泻下、抑菌、止血等作用的有效成分。经过炮制之后，具有泻下作用的成分降低，其泻下的副作用得以减轻。研究表明，具有泻下作用的成分结合型蒽醌在原药材中的含量为2.12%，在大黄片中的含量为2.11%，在酒大黄中含量为1.65%，熟大黄中含量为1.04%，大黄炭中含量为0.47%；而没有泻下作用的游离型蒽醌在原药材中的含量为1.35%，在大黄片中的含量为1.01%，在酒大黄中含量为1.43%，熟大黄中含量为1.50%，大黄炭中含量为2.60%。同时，具有止血作用的有效成分含量增加，具有抑菌作用的有效成分含量保持不变。

当　归

【来源】本品为伞形科植物当归的干燥根。

【炮制方法】

1. **当归**　取原药材，除去杂质，洗净，稍润，切薄片，晒干或低温干燥。

2. **酒当归**　取当归片，加入定量黄酒拌匀，稍闷润，待酒被吸尽后，置炒制容器内，用文火加热，炒至深黄色且表面有少许深色焦斑。每100kg当归片，用黄酒10kg。

3. **土炒当归**　将灶心土粉置预热过的炒制容器内，炒至灵活状态，倒入当归片，炒至当归片上粘满细土并逸出香气时，取出。每100kg当归片，用灶心土粉30kg。

4. **当归炭**　取当归片，置炒制容器内，用中火加热，炒至微黑色，质地松脆。

【炮制作用】

1. **当归**　具有补血、润肠通便的功能。如用于治疗血虚肠燥便秘的润肠丸。

2. **酒当归**　活血通经、祛瘀止痛的作用增强。适用于多种痛症，如经闭痛经，风湿痹痛，跌打损伤，瘀血肿痛。如用于治疗脓肿胀痛的仙方活命饮。

3. **土炒当归**　既能增强补血作用，又能缓和油润而不滑肠，可用于治疗血虚便溏。

4. **当归炭**　以补血止血为主，如用治妇人血崩的振阳丸。

【炮制研究】

由于所含成分有所不同，当归不同部位功效不同。当归头中挥发油含量较之当归尾低，因此具有更强的止血作用，当归尾行血作用较强，当归身则以养血为主，全药具有调节血液的作用。原药材中阿魏酸含量最高，多用于益气补血，缓急止痛。具有很强止血作用的单宁在当归炭中含量最高，如用于止血，当首选当归炭。

蕲　蛇

【来源】本品为蝰科动物五步蛇的干燥体。

【炮制方法】

1. **蕲蛇**　取原药材，除去头、鳞，切成寸段。

2. **蕲蛇肉**　取蕲蛇，去头，用定量黄酒润透后，除去鳞、骨，取净肉，干燥。每100kg蕲蛇段，用黄酒20kg。

3. **酒蕲蛇**　取蕲蛇段，加入定量黄酒拌匀，稍闷润，待酒被吸尽后，置炒制容器内，用文火加热，炒至黄色。每100kg蕲蛇段，用黄酒20kg。

【炮制作用】

1. **蕲蛇**　仅作外用，如用于皮肤瘙痒和惊厥。

2. **酒蕲蛇**　缓和药物腥臭之性，具有祛风除湿、通经止痛的作用。如用于治疗风湿痹痛的白花蛇酒；治疗卒中急风的蛇蝎续命汤。

【炮制目的】

1. 降低药物的毒性。

2. 对通经活络起到协同作用。

3. 提高药效成分的溶出率。

4. 矫臭矫味。

川 芎

【来源】本品为伞形科植物川芎的干燥根茎。

【炮制方法】

1. **川芎**　取原药材，除去杂质，洗净，润透，切薄片，干燥。

2. **酒川芎**　取川芎片，加入定量黄酒拌匀，稍闷润，待酒被吸尽后，置炒制容器内，用文火加热，炒至外表棕黄色，质地松脆。每 100kg 川芎片，用黄酒 10kg。

【炮制作用】

1. **川芎**　活血行气，祛风止痛。

2. **酒川芎**　使功效增加，增强活血行气止痛作用。如用治风邪头痛的川芎茶调散；治疗风湿头痛的羌活参石汤；治疗风热头痛的川芎散。

【炮制研究】

川芎中含有一种叫做川芎嗪的生物碱，其具有易升华的性质。为了避免这种有效成分的损失，药物的储存时间不能过长。

白 芍

【来源】本品为毛茛科植物芍药的干燥根。

【炮制方法】

1. **白芍**　取原药材，除去杂质，洗净，闷润至透，切薄片，干燥。

2. **酒白芍**　取白芍片，加入定量黄酒拌匀，稍闷润，待酒被吸尽后，置炒制容器内，用文火加热，炒至药物表面微黄色。每 100kg 白芍片，用黄酒 10kg。

3. **炒白芍**　取白芍片，置炒制容器内，用文火加热，炒至表面微黄色。

【炮制作用】

1. **白芍**　具有泻肝火、平抑肝阳、养阴除烦的功能。如用于镇肝息风汤和桂枝汤。

2. **酒白芍**　酸寒伐肝之性降低，具有调和脾胃、解痉的作用。用于胸胁疼痛等，如可用于逍遥散。

3. **炒白芍**　缓和药性，具有疏肝健脾、养血敛阴的作用。

【炮制研究】

白芍中含有多种有效成分。如具有镇痛、镇静和解痉作用的芍药苷；具有抗炎和抗血栓形成作用的芍药醇；具有解痉、镇痛和镇静作用的苯甲酸安替比林；具有抗炎作用的单宁。研究显示，白芍外皮中有效成分的含量为最高，因此临床使用中不去皮入药。由于单宁易被氧化，长时间储存或置于铁制容器中时，药物的颜色会由白色变为红色。

第二节 醋 炙 法

1. 定义

将净选或切制后的药物，加入定量米醋低温拌炒至规定程度的方法。

2. 目的

（1）引药入肝，增强活血理气止痛作用。如柴胡醋炙后能增强疏肝止痛的作用，延胡索醋炙后能增强活血散瘀的作用。

（2）降低毒性，缓和药性。如芫花经醋炙之后，可消减毒性，缓和峻下作用。

（3）矫臭矫味。如乳香经醋炙后可减少其不良气味。

（4）使药物易于粉碎和有效成分的溶出。如矿物药（自然铜）和贝类（龟甲）经过炮制之后，其质地由坚硬变为酥脆。

3. 工艺

醋制法有两种工艺。

（1）先拌醋后炒药。将净制或切制后的药物，加入定量米醋拌匀，闷润，待醋被吸尽后，置炒制容器内，用文火炒至一定程度，取出晾凉，即得。此法适用于大多数药物。

（2）先炒药后喷醋。将净选后的药物，置炒制容器内，文火炒至规定程度，喷洒定量米醋，炒至微干，取出后继续翻动，摊开晾凉。此法适用于树脂类、动物粪便类等容易相互黏结的药材。

4. 辅料用量

一般为每 100kg 药物，用米醋 20 ~ 30kg。

5. 适用药物

具有峻下逐水作用的药物（芫花）；具有疏肝理气作用的药物（柴胡）；具有活血化瘀作用的药物（延胡索）；具有不良气味的药物（乳香）。

柴 胡

【来源】本品为伞形科植物柴胡或狭叶柴胡的干燥根。

【炮制方法】

1. **柴胡** 取原药材，除去杂质及残茎，洗净，润透，切厚片，干燥。

2. **醋柴胡** 取柴胡片，加入定量的米醋拌匀，闷润至醋被吸尽，置炒制容器内，用文火加热，炒干。每 100kg 柴胡，用米醋 20kg。

3. **鳖血柴胡** 取柴胡片，加入定量洁净的新鲜鳖血及适量冷开水拌匀，闷润至鳖血液被吸尽，置炒制容器内，用文火加热，炒干。每 100kg 柴胡，用鳖血 13kg。

【炮制作用】

1. **柴胡** 升散作用较强，多用于解表退热，如用于小柴胡汤和补中益气汤。

2. **醋柴胡** 升散之性缓和，疏肝理气止痛作用增强，如用于逍遥散。

3. **鳖血柴胡** 填阴滋血，抑制其浮阳之性。可用于骨蒸劳热，发烧和疟疾。

【炮制研究】

柴胡中含有具有镇静、止痛、镇咳和解热作用的柴胡皂苷。醋炙之后在酸性条件下，柴胡皂苷能水解为具有止痛、镇咳和抗炎作用的柴胡皂苷元。同时，柴胡中具有解热作用的有效成分 α-菠菜甾醇在酸性条件下也将水解为酯类成分，其解热作用消失。因此，醋柴胡的主要功效不是解热，而是疏肝理气止痛。

延 胡 索

【来源】本品为罂粟科植物延胡索的干燥块茎。

【炮制方法】

1. **延胡索** 取原药材，洗净，润透，切厚片。

2. **醋炒延胡索** 取净延胡索，加入定量米醋拌匀，闷润至醋被吸尽后，置炒制容器内，用文火加热，炒干，取出晾凉。每100kg延胡索，用米醋20kg。

3. **醋煮延胡索** 取净延胡索，加入定量的米醋与适量清水（以平药面为宜），置煮制容器内，用文火加热煮至透心，取出，切厚片，晾干。每100kg延胡索，用米醋20kg。

4. **醋蒸延胡索** 取净延胡索，加入定量米醋拌匀，蒸至醋被吸尽，取出，切厚片，晾干。每100kg延胡索，用米醋20kg。

【炮制作用】

1. **延胡索** 很少应用。

2. **醋炙延胡索** 增强活血行气止痛的作用。如可用于乌金丸、延胡止痛片等。

【炮制研究】

延胡索经过炮制之后，止痛作用增强。第一是因为醋产生了协同作用（可增强对肝经的作用）；第二是因为延胡索中具有止痛作用的主要有效成分游离延胡索乙素经过醋炙之后可生成盐，增大有效成分在水中的溶出率。

研究显示，总生物碱在原药材中含量为25.06%，醋炙品中含量为49.33%，酒炙品中含量为22.66%。

此外，不同比例和种类的酸也可影响有效成分的溶出率。例如，炮制时使用酒石酸其有效成分的溶出率为68.02%，使用柠檬酸其有效成分溶出率为64.66%，都高于使用米醋。

乳 香

【来源】本品为橄榄科卡氏乳香树或鲍达乳香树皮部渗出的干燥胶树脂。

【炮制方法】

1. **乳香** 取原药材，除去杂质，将大块者砸碎。

2. **醋乳香** 取净乳香，置炒制容器内，用文火加热，炒至冒烟，表面微熔，喷淋定量米醋，边喷边炒至表面呈油亮光泽时，迅速取出，摊开放凉。每100kg乳香，用米醋 10kg。

3. 炒乳香 取净乳香，置炒制容器内，用文火加热，炒至冒烟，表面熔化显油亮光泽时，迅速取出，摊开放凉。

【炮制作用】

1. 乳香 对胃刺激性较强，易引起呕吐，只做外用。如用于制作九圣人散等。

2. 醋乳香 矫臭矫味，能协同增强活血止痛、收敛生肌的功效。

3. 炒乳香 能减少药物的刺激性，并使药物易于粉碎。

【炮制研究】

乳香中含有树脂、树胶和挥发油。其中含有树脂 60% ~ 70%，树胶 27% ~ 35%，经过醋炙之后，可除去大部分挥发油成分，减少刺激性。

芫　花

【来源】本品为瑞香科植物芫花的干燥花蕾。

【炮制方法】

1. 生芫花 取原药材，除去杂质及梗、叶。

2. 醋芫花 取净芫花，加入定量的米醋拌匀，闷润至醋被吸尽，置炒制容器内，用文火加热，炒至微干，取出干燥。每 100kg 芫花，加米醋 30kg。

3. 醋煮芫花 取净芫花，置煮制容器内，加入定量的米醋拌匀，煮至米醋被药物完全吸尽为度。每 100kg 芫花，加米醋 30 ~ 40kg 和水 30kg。

【炮制作用】

1. 生芫花 有毒。具有峻泻逐水之功效，仅做外用。如用于治疗牙痛的芫花散。

2. 醋芫花 毒性降低，缓和泻下作用，如用于舟车丸、十枣汤等。

【炮制目的】

1. 降低毒性。

2. 缓和泻下和腹痛症状。

【炮制研究】

芫花经过醋炙之后，在酸性条件下，芫花中的黄酮苷可水解为具有祛痰作用的芫花素。此外，具有刺激性的不饱和挥发性成分也发生了变化。研究显示，生芫花和醋芫花醇浸出物急性毒性试验中，LD_{50} 分别为 1.0% 和 17.78%；水浸出物急性毒性试验中，LD_{50} 分别为 8.3% 和 7.07%。结果显示，芫花经过炮制之后毒性降低。

第三节　盐炙法

1. 定义

将净选或切制后的药物，加入一定量食盐水溶液用文火拌炒的方法。

2. 目的

（1）盐炙能引药入肾。例如，杜仲的主要功效为补肝肾，强筋骨，安胎。盐炙后可引药入肾经并增强其功效。

（2）盐炙可增强药效。例如，黄柏的主要作用为泻火解毒，清热燥湿。经过盐炙之后，可缓和苦燥之性，并可引药入肾经以泻肾火。

（3）缓和药性。例如，盐炙可以缓和补骨脂的辛燥之性。

3. 工艺

盐炙法有两种工艺。

（1）先拌盐水后炒。适用于大多数药物。

将药物与食盐水混合均匀，放置闷润，置炒制容器内，用文火炒至盐水被吸尽，取出晾凉。

（2）先炒药后加盐水。适用于含黏液质较多的药物，如车前子。

先将药物置炒制容器内，用文火炒至一定程度，再喷淋盐水，炒干，取出晾凉。

4. 加辅料量

通常每100kg药物，用食盐2kg，水8~10kg。

5. 适用药物

多用于补肾固精、疗疝、利尿和泻相火的药物。

车 前 子

【来源】本品为车前科植物车前或平车前的干燥成熟种子。

【炮制方法】

1. 车前子 取原药材，除去杂质。

2. 盐车前子 取净车前子，置炒制容器内，用文火加热，炒至略有爆鸣声时，喷淋盐水，炒干，取出晾凉。

3. 炒车前子 取净车前子，置炒制容器内，用文火加热，炒至略有爆声，并有香气逸出时，取出晾凉。

【炮制作用】

1. 车前子 味甘，性寒，具有清热利尿、渗湿通淋的功能，如用于水肿胀满、热淋涩痛等症的车前子散。

2. 盐车前子 补肝肾，增强视力，减轻水肿。如用治肝肾俱虚、眼昏目暗的驻景丸。

3. 炒车前子 缓和寒凉之性，渗湿而不伤脾，如用于治疗因脾虚而引起渗湿止泻的四苓散。

【炮制研究】

车前子经过盐炙之后，黄酮类成分含量发生改变，有效成分溶出率提高。研究显示，有效成分的溶出率在车前子生品中含量为71.32%，盐炙品中含量为81%，清炒品中含量为84.70%。

黄 柏

【来源】本品为芸香科植物黄树皮的干燥树皮。

【炮制方法】

1. **黄柏**　取原药材，除去杂质，刮去残留的粗皮，洗净，润透，切丝或块，干燥。

2. **盐黄柏**　取黄柏丝或块，用盐水拌匀，稍闷，待盐水被吸尽后，置炒制容器内，用文火加热，炒至外表呈深黄色有焦斑。每100kg药物，用食盐2kg。

3. **酒黄柏**　取黄柏丝或块，用黄酒拌匀，稍闷，待酒被吸尽后，置炒制容器内，用文火加热，炒干，且外表呈淡黄色，逸出酒香。每100kg药物，用黄酒10kg。

4. **黄柏炭**　取黄柏丝或块，置炒制容器内，用武火加热，炒至表面焦黑色，内部深褐色。

【炮制作用】

1. **黄柏**　具有泻火解毒、清热燥湿的功能。如治湿热痢疾的白头翁汤；治伤寒身黄、发热的栀子柏皮汤。

2. **盐黄柏**　缓和苦燥之性，可引药入肾经，清泻相火。如治阴虚骨蒸、盗汗、遗精的大补阴丸。

3. **酒黄柏**　增强药效，缓和药物苦寒之性，善清上焦湿热。如治目赤、咽喉肿痛的上清丸。

4. **黄柏炭**　味苦、性涩，具有清热止血的作用，多用于便血、崩漏下血。

黄柏除了以上四种炮制方法以外，还可进行蜜炙，可用于治疗口腔溃疡。

【炮制研究】

黄柏经过水处理之后其小檗碱含量会发生变化。为了避免有效成分的流失，在净制和切制过程中应抢水洗并及时切成块。此外，黄柏经过炮制之后，小檗碱含量也会发生变化。研究显示，在黄柏原药材、酒炙品、盐炙品和炭品中小檗碱含量分别为100%、96%、87%和16%。

杜　仲

【来源】本品为杜仲科植物杜仲的干燥树皮。

【炮制方法】

1. **杜仲**　取原药材，刮去粗皮，洗净，润透，切丝或块。

2. **盐杜仲**　取杜仲丝或块，加盐水拌匀，稍闷，待盐水被吸尽后，置炒制容器内，用中火炒至颜色加深，有焦斑，丝易断时，取出晾凉。每100kg杜仲丝或块，用食盐2kg。

【炮制作用】

1. **杜仲**　具有补肝肾、强筋骨、安胎的作用。

2. **盐杜仲**　盐炙引药入肾，补肝肾、强筋骨、安胎的作用增强。如治疗肾虚腰痛的青娥丸，治疗高血压症的杜仲降压片。

【炮制研究】

研究显示，杜仲原药材和盐炙品中有效成分的比例分别为10.37%和18.44%。药理试验表明，盐杜仲比生品具有更强的降压作用。

第四节 姜炙法

1. 定义

将净选或切制后的药物，加入定量姜汁用文火加热拌炒至一定程度的方法。

2. 目的

（1）缓和药性。例如，黄连姜炙可制其过于苦寒之性，使药性缓和。

（2）增强和胃止呕作用。例如，黄连经过姜炙之后可增强止呕作用，砂仁经过姜炙可增强温胃止呕的功效，而竹茹姜炙长于降逆止呕。

（3）减少刺激性。例如，厚朴对咽喉有一定的刺激性，姜炙可缓和其刺激性，并能增强温中化湿除胀的功效；半夏生品具有刺激性，经过姜炙之后，刺激性降低，并能增强其降逆止呕的作用。

3. 工艺

姜炙法有两种炮制工艺。

（1）先加辅料后炒。此方法从新鲜生姜榨取或研磨得到姜汁，或者以干姜煎汁。

将药物与一定量的姜汁拌匀，放置闷润，使姜汁逐渐深入药物内部。置炒制容器内，用文火炒至一定程度，取出晾凉。

（2）姜汤煮。将鲜姜片煎汤，加入药物煮两小时，待姜汁基本被吸尽，取出，进行干燥，切片。

4. 加辅料量

每100kg药物，用生姜10kg或干姜10/3kg。

5. 适用药物

多用于祛痰止咳、降逆止呕的药物。

厚 朴

【来源】本品为木兰科植物厚朴或凹叶厚朴的干燥干皮、根皮及枝皮。

【炮制方法】

1. **厚朴** 取原药材，刮去粗皮，洗净，润透，切丝，干燥。

2. **姜厚朴** 取厚朴丝，加姜汁拌匀，闷润，待姜汁被吸尽后，置炒制容器内，用文火加热，炒干。

3. **姜汁煮厚朴** 取生姜切片，加水煮汤，另取刮尽粗皮的药材，扎成捆，置姜汤中，反复浇淋，并用微火加热共煮，至姜液被吸尽时取出，切丝，干燥。每100kg厚朴，用生姜10kg或干姜10/3kg。

【炮制作用】

1. **厚朴** 具有燥湿消痰、下气除满的功能，对咽喉具有刺激性，故内服一般不生用。

2. **姜厚朴** 消除对咽喉的刺激性，并可增强宽中和胃的功效。如治湿滞脾胃的平胃散。

【炮制目的】

1. 减少刺激性。

2. 增强协同作用，增强疗效。

【炮制研究】

厚朴净制去粗皮的目的是提高其有效成分的相对含量。厚朴中厚朴酚、和厚朴酚具有抗菌、镇静和抗胃溃疡的作用；挥发油具有镇静、发汗、祛痰和平喘作用。经过姜炙之后，以上成分含量均有所增加或发生变化。

竹 茹

【来源】本品为禾本科植物青秆竹、大头典竹或淡竹茎秆的干燥中间层。

【炮制方法】

1. **竹茹** 取原药材，除去杂质和硬皮，切断或揉成小团。

2. **姜竹茹** 取竹茹段或团，加姜汁拌匀，稍润，待姜汁被吸尽后，置炒制容器内，用文火加热，如烙饼法将两面烙至微黄色，取出晾凉。每100kg竹茹，用生姜10kg。

【炮制作用】

1. **竹茹** 具有清肺化痰的作用，用于肺热咯血等症的治疗。

2. **姜竹茹** 增强降逆止呕的功效，如治疗胃虚有热，呕逆的橘皮竹茹汤。

第五节 蜜 炙 法

1. 定义

将净选或切制后的药物，加入一定量炼蜜用文火拌炒至一定程度的方法。蜜炙法所使用的蜂蜜都要先加热炼过。

2. 目的

（1）增加药物有效性的作用。如百部蜜炙后能增强润肺止咳的作用。黄芪原药材的主要作用是益气固表，蜜炙能起到协同作用，增强其补中益气的功效。

（2）缓和药性。例如，马兜铃生品味苦、性寒，具有清肺降气、止咳平喘的功能，经过蜜炙之后，能缓和其药性，并增强润肺止咳的功效。麻黄生品具有发汗解表的功效，经过蜜炙之后，缓和了辛散发汗的作用，以宣肺平喘力胜。

（3）矫味和消除副作用。例如，马兜铃生品易致恶心呕吐，经过蜜炙之后，能矫正其不良气味，并减少呕吐的副作用。

3. 工艺

蜜炙法有两种炮制工艺。

（1）先拌蜜后炒药。适用于质地酥脆的药物。

先取一定量的炼蜜，加适量开水稀释，与药物拌匀，放置闷润，使蜜逐渐渗入药物组织内部，然后置预热的锅内，用文火炒至颜色加深、不黏手时，取出摊晾。

（2）先炒药后加蜜。适用于质地致密的药物。

先将药物置预热的锅内，用文火炒至颜色加深时，再加入一定量的炼蜜，迅速翻动，使蜜与药物拌匀，炒至不黏手，取出摊晾。

4. 加辅料量

通常为每100kg 药物，用炼蜜25kg。

5. 适用药物

多用于止咳平喘、补脾益气的药物。

6. 注意事项

（1）炼蜜若过于浓稠，可加适量开水稀释。

（2）炼蜜必须与药物充分拌匀闷润，使蜜完全渗入药物组织内部。

（3）蜜炙时，火力一定要小，以免焦化。

（4）蜜炙药物须凉后密闭贮存，并放置阴凉处，不宜受日光直接照射。

甘 草

【来源】本品为豆科植物甘草的干燥根及根茎。

【炮制方法】

1. **甘草** 取原药材，除去杂质，洗净，润透，切厚片，晒干。

2. **蜜甘草** 取炼蜜，加适量开水稀释后，淋入净甘草片中拌匀，闷润，置炒制容器内，用文火加热，炒至老黄色、不黏手时，取出晾凉。每100kg 甘草片，用炼蜜25kg。

【炮制作用】

1. **甘草** 长于泻火解毒、化痰止咳。例如，可用于治疗疮疡的茵华甘草汤，治疗热痰咳嗽的沙参麦冬汤，治疗咽喉肿痛的桔梗汤。

2. **蜜甘草** 以补中益气、缓急止痛力胜。如用于四君子汤和炙甘草汤。

【炮制研究】

甘草根具有保护黏膜以缓解咳嗽的作用以及良好的解毒效果。其产生解毒作用的主要原因为：①具有类肾上腺素作用；②提高肝脏的解毒功能；③帮助吸附有毒成分；④甘草酸所分解成的葡萄糖醛酸可与有毒成分相结合。

研究表明，甘草切制前的软化处理，以水浸泡48 小时的水溶出物损耗率为49.89%，以水浸润48 小时则为7.22%，甘草酸损耗率分别是48.40% 和4.99%。饮片厚度也会影响甘草酸的浸出率，如当饮片厚度为2~3mm 时，其浸出率为99.91%，饮片厚度为5~

6mm 时，浸出率为 85.22%。

麻　黄

【来源】本品为麻黄科植物草麻黄、中麻黄或木贼麻黄的干燥草质茎。

【炮制方法】

1. **麻黄**　取原药材，除去木质茎、残根及杂质，稍润，切断，干燥。

2. **蜜麻黄**　取炼蜜，加适量开水稀释，淋入麻黄段中拌匀，闷润，置炒制容器内，用文火加热，炒至不黏手时，取出晾凉。每 100kg 麻黄段，用炼蜜 20kg。

3. **麻黄绒**　取麻黄段，碾绒，筛去粉末。

4. **蜜麻黄绒**　取炼蜜，加适量开水稀释，淋入麻黄绒内拌匀，闷润，置炒制容器内，用文火加热，炒至深黄色、不黏手时，取出晾凉。每 100kg 麻黄绒，用炼蜜 25kg。

【炮制作用】

1. **麻黄**　具有发汗散寒、宣肺平喘、利水消肿的功能，如用于治疗外感风寒，表实无汗的麻黄汤；治疗风水证，恶风，面目浮肿的越婢汤。

2. **蜜麻黄**　辛散发汗作用缓和，以宣肺平喘力胜。如用于治疗表证较轻，而肺气雍闭的三拗汤。

3. **麻黄绒**　辛散发表作用更缓和，具有利水消肿的功效。用于老人及小儿风寒感冒。

4. **蜜麻黄绒**　止咳平喘。适用于表证已解而咳喘未愈的患者。

【炮制研究】

经过炮制之后，麻黄中生物碱含量变化不大，挥发油成分含量减少，麻黄根与茎在临床使用中功效有所不同。

第六节　油　炙　法

1. 定义

将净选或切制后的药物，与一定量的食用油脂共同加热处理的方法。

2. 目的

（1）增强药物温肾助阳的作用。

（2）利于粉碎，便于制剂和服用。

3. 工艺

油炙法有三种炮制工艺。

（1）油炒。取药物与油充分拌匀，置炒制容器内，用文火快速炒至油被吸尽。每 100kg 药物，用油 20kg。

（2）油炸。将油倒入锅内加热，至沸腾时，倾入药物，用文火炸至药物酥脆为度。每 100kg 药物，用油 25kg。

（3）油烤。药物切成块放炉火上烤热，用油涂布，加热烘烤，待油渗入药内后，再涂再烤，反复操作，直至药物质地酥脆。

淫 羊 藿

【来源】本品为小檗科植物淫羊藿、箭叶淫羊藿、柔毛淫羊藿或朝鲜淫羊藿的干燥叶。

【炮制方法】

1. **淫羊藿**　取原药材，除去杂质，稍润，切丝，干燥。

2. **炙淫羊藿**　取羊脂油置锅内加热熔化，加入淫羊藿丝，用文火加热，炒至微黄色，油脂吸尽，微显光泽时，取出。每100kg淫羊藿，用炼油20kg。

【炮制作用】

1. **淫羊藿**　祛风湿，强筋骨，如用于淫羊藿散和淫羊藿丸。

2. **炙淫羊藿**　补肾助阳。如用于治疗肾气衰弱的三肾丸。

蛤 蚧

【来源】本品为壁虎科动物蛤蚧除去内脏的干燥全体。

【炮制方法】

1. **蛤蚧**　取原药材，除去竹片，洗净，除去头和足爪及鳞片，切成小块，干燥。

2. **酒蛤蚧**　取蛤蚧块，用黄酒拌匀，闷润，待酒被吸尽后，置炒制容器内，用文火炒干。每100kg蛤蚧块，用黄酒20kg。

3. **油酥蛤蚧**　取蛤蚧，涂以麻油，用无烟火烤至稍黄质脆，切成小块。

【炮制作用】

1. **蛤蚧**　具有补肺益肾、纳气定喘、助阳益精的功效。

2. **酒炙蛤蚧**　增强了补肾壮阳的功效。

3. **油酥蛤蚧**　功效与生品相同，酥制后易粉碎，腥气减少。

Chapter Ten   Calcining Method

1. Definition

The method of calcining drugs with direct fire.

2. Classification

Three types of methods include calcining openly, calcining and quenching, and hermetic calcining.

3. Suitable Drugs

The method of calcining with direct fire is suitable for drugs of mineral, shellfish and fossil. The calcining and quenching method is suitable for mineral drugs with harder texture or drugs for special needs in clinical applications, the method of hermetic calcining is suitable for drugs that are easy to be ashed in charring.

4. Notice

(1) Drugs' inherent nature should be kept after being calcined. For example, the method of hermetic calcining can be used in processing some plant drugs to avoid being ashed.

(2) Drugs should be separated by size to avoid unevenness in the processing degree.

(3) Drugs should be ground into powders for clinical applications.

Section One   Calcining with Direct Fire

1. Definition

It means calcining with direct fire.

2. Purposes

(1) Strengthen effects. For example, after being calcined, the effect of warming the kidney to invigorate *yang* of Stalactitum (*Zhongrushi*) would be strengthened.

(2) Change drugs' nature and effects. For example, the main effects of raw product of Gypsum Fibrosum (*Shigao*) are to clear heat and purge away pathogenic fire, relieve restlessness and thirst. After being calcined, the main effects of dried Gypsum are to arrest dampness and ulceration to stop bleeding.

(3) Reduce toxicity. For example, after being calcined, the main effects of Ophicalcitum (*Huaruishi*) are to moderate acidity, impair spleen and stomach. The great cold nature of Calcitum (*Hanshuishi*) could also be moderated.

3. Operating Methods

(1) Direct method. Put drugs in heater or fire, calcine thoroughly until the drugs become flaming red inside and take them out of the container. Crush when used in clinic.

(2) Indirect method. Put drugs in a refractory container, then put the container in a heater or over fire, and calcine thoroughly until the drugs become flaming red inside. Crush when used in clinic.

4. Notice

(1) Calcine thoroughly without stirring.

(2) Choose suitable time and temperature.

(3) Avoid exploding and spilling when calcining.

(4) Store after drugs being cool.

Gypsum Fibrosum (Shigao)

【Source】 Sulfates minerals, hydrated calcium sulfate ($CaSO_4 \cdot 2H_2O$) .

【Processing Methods】

1. Raw Gypsum Fibrosum　Clean and dry under the sun, beat drugs into small pieces, or grind them into powder.

2. Calcining Gypsum Fibrosum　Put drugs in a refractory container, then put the container in heater or over strong fire, and calcine thoroughly until the drugs become flaming red inside . Crush when used in clinical applications.

【Processing Functions】

1. Raw Gypsum Fibrosum　It can clear heat and purge away pathogenic fire. It can also relieve restlessness and thirst. For example, it can be used in Baihu Decoction, which is suitable for high fever, restlessness and thirst. It can also be used in Maxing Shigan decoction, which is suitable for cough and asthma due to lung – heat.

2. Calcined Gypsum Fibrosum　It arrests dampness and ulceration to stop bleeding.

【Processing Research】

For the raw Gypsum Fibrosum, the main effect is clearing away heat. After being calcined, the dried Gypsum's effect of releasing heat is moderated while its main effect lies in astringing, which results from the change of contents. In the process of heating, Gypsum Fibrosum would lose two water molecules and the astringent effect would be strengthened.

Alumen (Baifan)

【Source】 Sulfate minerals, potassium aluminium sulfate containing water [KAl (SO$_4$)$_2$ · 12H$_2$O] .

【Processing Methods】

1. Raw Alumen   Remove impurities, pound into pieces or grind into powder.

2. Calcining Alumen   Put clean Alumen in a refractory container, then put the container in a heater and heat it with strong fire until the drugs melt, calcine until drugs expand and become white honeycomb – shaped solid, then take drugs out and get them cold, and crush when used in clinical applications.

Alumen is semitransparent and has hard texture. After being calcined, dried alum shows a white honeycomb without cluster and has crisp texture. During calcining, stirring is forbidden.

【Processing Functions】

1. Raw Alumen   It has sour and cold nature, which can relieve internal heat and kill worms. It clears away heat and disperses phlegm, and deprives the wetness to alleviate itching. For example, it can be used in Platinum Pill which is suitable for epilepsy due to wind – phlegm.

2. Calcined Alumen   The sour and cold nature is moderated. It can alleviate vomiting, cause contraction and arrest discharge, treat ulceration and stop bleeding and suppration. For example, it can be used in Promote Tissue Regeneration Powder which is suitable for ulcerous nonunion.

【Processing Research】

After being calcined, the main effect of alum is to treat ulceration through diminishing effusion and form precipitation after the contents combine with protein of blood plasma.

Os Draconis (Longgu)

【Source】 Mammalian skeleton fossil from ancient times.

【Processing Methods】

1. Raw Os Draconis   Remove impurities.

2. Calcining Os Draconis   Put drugs in a refractory container, then put the container in a heater or over fire. High heat is used during processing until the drugs' color transforms from white – yellow to taupe color.

【Processing Functions】

1. Raw Os Draconis   It can relieve convulsion and check exuberant *yang*. For example, it can be used in Zhenxin Dingxian Decoction which is suitable for convulsive epilepsy.

2. Calcined Os Draconis   It can cause contraction and arrest discharge, and promote tissue regeneration. For example, it can be used in Longgu Powder which is suitable for chronic metrorrhagia.

Concha Ostreae （Muli）

【Source】 The shell of oyster.

【Processing Methods】

1. Raw Concha Ostreae　Clean and dry under the sun, then grind drugs to powder.

2. Calcining Concha Ostreae　Put drugs in heater or over fire, calcine thoroughly until the drugs become crisp and take them out of the container. Crush when used in clinical applications.

【Processing Functions】

1. Raw Concha Ostreae　A tranquilizer, it has the function of checking exuberant *yang* and nourishing *yin*, softening hard lumps and dispelling nodes. Be used for crewels and scrofula, phlegm nodule.

2. Calcinied Concha Ostreae　It can cause contraction and arrest discharge. For example, it can be used in Muli Powder which is suitable for treating night sweat and spontaneous perspiration.

Section Two　Calcining and Quenching

1. Definition

After being calcined thoroughly the drugs are added into a quenching liquid as soon as possible to get the drugs cool suddenly. The quenching liquids include water, vinegar, wine or drugs' juice.

2. Purposes

（1） Make drugs' texture crisper and easy to be crushed, which is good for decocting of the effective ingredients.

（2） Change drugs' physico-chemical properties, while reduce side-effects and strengthen drugs' effects.

（3） Reduce toxicity and remove foreign materials.

3. Operating Methods

Put drugs in heater or over fire, calcine thoroughly until the drugs become flaming red inside and take drugs out of container. Then put drugs into quenching liquid quickly. Repeat the procedure several times if needed until drugs' texture becomes crisper.

4. Notice

（1） Drugs processed by this method should be calcined and quenched repeatedly.

（2）If the quenching liquid is vinegar, wine or drugs' juice, they should be absorbed thoroughly by drugs.

（3）Choose suitable quenching liquids according to processing purpose and drugs' nature.

Pyritum（Zirantong）

【Source】 Iron disulfide. Mainly contain FeS_2.

【Processing Methods】

1. Raw Pyritum　Clean and dry under the sun, then pound drugs to small pieces.

2. Calcining and quenching Pyritum　Put drugs in a heater or over fire, calcine thoroughly until the drugs become red inside and take drugs out of container. Put drugs into vinegar quickly. Repeat the procedure of calcining and quenching for several times until drugs' texture become crisper. 30kg vinegar per 100kg drugs.

【Processing Functions】

1. Raw Pyritum　It can eliminate stasis to activate blood circulation, set bones and stop pain.

2. Calcined and quenched Pyritum　Drugs' texture become crisper and easier to decoct effective components. The effects of eliminating stasis to activate blood circulation, and relieving pain would be strengthened.

【Processing Research】

The reasons for the strengthening of effects lie in the change of contents. After being processed, the iron disulfide would generate iron sulfide which could react with acetic acid in vinegar to produce ferrous acetate. Bivalence ferrous ions are easy to be absorbed by body, which would inevitably enhance the effect of eliminating stasis to activate blood circulation and relieving pain.

Haematitum（Daizheshi）

【Source】 Oxydum haematite. Mainly contain Fe_2O_3.

【Processing Methods】

1. Raw Haematitum　Clean and dry under the sun, then break drugs into small pieces.

2. Calcining and quenching Haematitum　Put drugs in a heater or over strong fire, calcine thoroughly until the drugs become red inside and take drugs out of container. Put drugs into vinegar quickly. Repeat the procedure of calcining and quenching for several times until drugs' texture become crisper. 30kg vinegar per 100kg drugs.

【Processing Functions】

1. Raw Haematitum　It can pacify liver and subdue *yang*, check upward perverted flow of *qi* and cool the blood and stanch bleeding. For example, it can be used in Liver – Wind Suppressing Decoction.

2. Calcinied and quenchied Haematitum　It can moderate the bitter and cold nature, and calm the liver and stanch bleeding. Be used for empsyxis, haematemesis, metrorrhagia and metrostaxis.

【Processing Research】

After being processed, ferric ion is deoxidized to bivalence iron which is easy to be absorbed by the stomach, which can strengthen the effects of the drugs.

Calamine (Luganshi)

【Source】 Carbonate mineral. Mainly contain $ZnCO_3$.

【Processing Methods】

1. Raw Calamine　Remove impurities.

2. Calcining and quenching Calamine　Put drugs in a heater or over fire, calcine thoroughly until the drugs become flaming red inside and take drugs out of container. Add drugs into water quickly. Quench and stir drugs in water and pour the upper suspension to a beaker or other similar container, repeat the procedure of calcining and quenching for 3 ~ 4 times. Put the upper suspension together, let it stand for hours then pour clear supernatant and collect precipitate, make them dry.

3. Processing Calamine　Add drugs' juice to the fine powder of the calcined and quenched calamine then mix thoroughly and dry. The drugs' juice includes Coptidis Rhizoma, Sanhuang (Coptidis Rhizome, Cortex Phellodendri and Radix Scutellariae) or Wuhuang (Coptidis Rhizome, Cortex Phellodendri, Radix Scutellariae, Fructus Gardeniae and Radix et Rhizoma Rhei) juice. 12.5kg adjuvant drugs per 100kg calcined and quenched Calamine.

【Processing Functions】

1. Raw Calamine　It is less used in clinical applications.

2. Calcinied and quenched Calamine　It is pure and exquisite, which is suitable for ophthalmology and external applications.

3. Processed Calamine　It can clear heat and improve eyesight, healing sores and eliminate dampness.

Section Three　Hermetic Calcining

1. Definition

It means calcining drugs to a carbonized state at a high temperature without oxygen.

2. Purposes

(1) Produce or strengthen hemostasis effect, for example, Crinis Carbonisatus (*Xueyutan*), Petiolus Trachycarpi Carbonisatus (*Zonglütan*).

(2) Reduce toxicity, for example, Resina Toxicodendri (*Ganqi*), Nidus Vespae (*Fengfang*).

3. Operating Methods

Put drugs in a big pot with a small pot covered with weights. Be closed by brine sludge or sand and calcined with high temperature.

4. Notice

（1） Char but without ashing.

（2） During processing, suitable amounts should be used to avoid charring unevenly.

（3） Open the pot after drugs are thoroughly cool.

5. Methods for inspection of hermetic calcining finished

（1） Water boils as soon as it drips on the bottom of the covered small pot.

（2） The paper on the bottom of the covered small pot transforms from white to yellow.

（3） The rice on the bottom of the covered small pot transforms from white to yellow.

（4） The color of smoke from fissure transforms from black to white during processing.

Crinis Carbonisatus （Xueyutan）

【Source】 Human hair.

【Processing Methods】

1. Hair　Remove impurities, and clean with caustic soda, then rinse and dry under the sun.

2. Crinis Carbonisatus　Put cleaned hair in a big pot with a small pot covered with weights. The pots are closed by brine sludge or sand, and calcined with high temperature.

【Processing Functions】

Produce new drugs with hemostasis effect. The drugs can be used in Bleeding – Stopping Pills which is suitable for all kinds of hemorrhages in the clinical applications.

【Processing Research】

The components in hair include brinolase, fat, iron, zinc, copper, calcium and magnesium. After being processed, the contents of calcium and iron are increased which will also strengthen the effects of hemostasis. Pharmacological test also shows that Crinis Carbonisatus could shorten clotting time and shrink blood vessels.

Trachycarpi Petiolus （Zonglü）

【Source】 Dry leafstalk of.

【Processing Methods】

1. Raw Trachycarpi Petiolus　Remove impurities, and cut drugs into sections.

2. Hermetic Calcining Trachycarpi Petiolus　Put drugs in a big pot with a small pot covered with weights. The pots are closed by brine sludge or sand and calcined with high temperature.

3. Charring Trachycarpi Petiolus　Preheat a pot with a high heat, fry quickly until drugs' outer part shows black brown color.

【Processing Functions】

1. **Raw Trachycarpi petiolus**   Do not use it when it is raw.

2. **Crinis Trachycarpi**   It has the function of stanching bleeding. For example, it can be used in Wujin Powder which is suitable for metrorrhagia.

Resina Toxicodendri (Ganqi)

【Source】 Resin of Toxicoden dron vernicifluum (Stokes) F. A. Barkl.

【Processing Methods】

1. **Hermetic Calcining Resina Toxicodendri**   Put drugs in a big pot with a small pot covered with weights. The pots are closed by brine sludge or sand and calcined with high temperature.

2. **Stir – frying Resina Toxicodendri**   Preheat a pot with a high heat, fry quickly until drugs' outer part is burnt, then dry until there is no smoke.

【Processing Functions】

1. **Hermetic Calcinied Resina Toxicodendri**   Do not use it when it is raw.

2. **Stir – fried Resina Toxicodendri**   It can reduce toxicity and irritation, activate stagnated blood and remove food retention, and kill worms. For example, it can be used in Ganqi Powder which is suitable for inactive extravasated blood.

【Processing Research】

The component in Resina Toxicodendri which is called urushiol would cause sensitization dermatitis. After being calcined, the content of the component would be reduced, the irritation would be moderated, and the effect of shortening bleeding and clotting time would be enhanced.

第十章 煅 法

1. 定义

直接用火煅烧的方法。

2. 分类

煅法分为明煅法、煅淬法、闷煅法。

3. 适用药物

煅法主要适用于矿物类中药，以及质地坚硬的贝壳类、化石类药物。煅淬法适用于质地坚硬的矿物药，以及临床上因特殊需要而必须煅淬的药物。闷煅法适用于炒炭易灰化的制炭药物。

4. 注意事项

（1）煅制药物时，要达到煅至"存性"的质量要求。例如，用闷煅法煅制一些植物类药材。
（2）药物必须大小分档，以免煅制时生熟不均。
（3）临床应用时，药物可磨成粉末。

第一节 明 煅 法

1. 定义

直火煅法。

2. 明煅法的目的

（1）增强药效。例如，钟乳石经明煅后温肾壮阳作用增强。
（2）改变药物的性质和药效。例如，生石膏具有清热泻火、除烦止渴的功效。经明煅后的煅石膏则具有收湿、敛疮止血的功能。
（3）降低毒性。例如，花蕊石煅后能缓和酸涩之性，消除伤脾伐胃的作用。寒水石煅后降低大寒之性。

3. 操作方法

（1）直接煅法。将药物直接加热或煅烧，煅至红透后取出。临床使用时粉碎。

（2）间接煅法。将药物置于耐火容器中再放入炉火中加热，煅至红透。临床使用时粉碎。

4. 注意事项

（1）煅至完全且煅制过程中不能搅拌。

（2）煅制温度、时间要适度。

（3）煅制过程中以防爆溅。

（4）药物彻底凉透后储存。

石　膏

【来源】本品为硫酸盐类矿物，主要含含水硫酸钙（$CaSO_4 \cdot 2H_2O$）。

【炮制方法】

1. 生石膏　取原药材，洗净，晒干，敲成小块，碾成细粉。

2. 煅石膏　取净石膏块置耐火容器内，用武火加热，煅至红透。使用时碾碎。

【炮制作用】

1. 生石膏　具有清热泻火、除烦止渴的功效。如治高热烦渴的白虎汤；治肺热咳喘的麻杏石甘汤。

2. 煅石膏　具收湿、敛疮止血的功效。

【炮制研究】

生石膏有明显的解热作用。而煅石膏解热作用减弱，主要作用在于收敛。原因在于成分的变化。石膏加热过程中失去两分子水后收敛作用增强。

白　矾

【来源】本品为硫酸盐类矿物，主含含水硫酸铝钾［$KAl(SO_4)_2 \cdot 12H_2O$］。

【炮制方法】

1. 白矾　取原药材，除去杂质，捣碎或研细。

2. 枯矾　取净白矾，置耐火容器内，用武火加热至熔化，继续煅至膨胀松泡呈白色蜂窝状固体，放凉取出，使用时研细。

白矾半透明、质地坚硬。枯矾呈白色、蜂窝状，质松易碎。煅制过程中不得搅拌。

【炮制作用】

1. 白矾　味酸、性寒，解毒、杀虫，并具有清热消痰、燥湿止痒的功能。如治风痰壅盛所致癫痫的白金丸。

2. 枯矾　酸寒之性降低，涌吐作用减弱，增强了收涩敛疮、止血化腐作用。如治疗疮口不合的生肌散。

【炮制研究】

白矾煅枯后，能和蛋白质反应生成难溶于水的物质而沉淀，减少疮面的渗出物而起生肌保护作用。

龙　骨

【来源】本品为古代哺乳动物骨骼类化石。

【炮制方法】

1. **龙骨**　取原药材，除去灰屑与杂质。

2. **煅龙骨**　取净龙骨小块，置耐火容器内，用武火加热，煅制药物由浅黄色变为灰褐色。

【炮制作用】

1. **龙骨**　镇惊潜阳作用较强。如治惊痫的镇心定痫汤。

2. **煅龙骨**　增强收敛固涩、生肌的功效。如治血崩不止的龙骨散。

牡　蛎

【来源】本品为牡蛎科动物的贝壳。

【炮制方法】

1. **牡蛎**　取原药材，洗净，晒干，碾碎。

2. **煅牡蛎**　取净牡蛎，置耐火容器内，用武火加热，煅至酥脆时取出，使用时碾碎。

【炮制作用】

1. **牡蛎**　具有重镇安神、潜阳补阴、软坚散结的功能。用于治瘰疬痰核。

2. **煅牡蛎**　增强了收敛固涩的作用。如用于盗汗自汗的牡蛎散。

第二节　煅淬法

1. 定义

将药物按明煅法煅至红透后，立即投入规定的液体辅料中骤然冷却的方法称煅淬。常用的淬液有水、醋、酒或药汁。

2. 煅淬的目的

（1）使药物质地酥脆，易于粉碎，利于有效成分煎出。

（2）改变药物的理化性质，减少副作用，增强疗效。

（3）消除毒性、清除杂质。

3. 操作方法

将药物按明煅法煅至红透后取出，立即投入液体辅料中。反复多次直至药物质脆易碎。

4. 注意事项

（1）药物煅淬一般要反复多次。

（2）煅淬时药物要吸尽醋、酒、药汁等淬液。

（3）根据各药物的性质和煅淬目的要求淬液种类和用量。

自　然　铜

【来源】本品为硫化物类矿物，主含二硫化铁（FeS_2）。

【炮制方法】

自然铜　取原药材，除去杂质，洗净，晒干，砸碎。

煅自然铜　取净自然铜，置耐火容器内，用武火加热，煅至红透后取出，立即投入醋中淬制。反复多次醋淬至质地酥脆。每100kg自然铜，用醋30kg。

【炮制作用】

1. **自然铜**　具有散瘀、接骨、止痛的作用。

2. **煅自然铜**　煅淬后质地变疏松，有效成分易于煎出。散瘀止痛作用增强。

【炮制研究】

药效增强的主要原因在于成分发生了变化。自然铜经火煅后二硫化铁分解为硫化铁，经醋淬后表面又生成醋酸铁，这使药物中铁离子溶出增加，更利于体内吸收，故增强了散瘀止痛的作用。

代　赭　石

【来源】本品为氧化物类矿物石，主含三氧化二铁（Fe_2O_3）。

【炮制方法】

1. **代赭石**　取原药材，除去杂质，洗净晒干，砸碎。

2. **煅赭石**　取净赭石，置耐火容器内，用武火加热，煅至红透后取出，立即投入醋中淬制。反复多次醋淬至质地酥脆。每100kg自然铜，用醋30kg。

【炮制作用】

1. **代赭石**　具有平肝潜阳、重镇降逆、凉血止血的功能。如用于肝风抑止汤。

2. **煅赭石**　降低了苦寒之性，增强了平肝止血功能。用于吐血、衄血、崩漏等症。

【炮制研究】

代赭石经煅淬后比生品亚铁含量增高，更利于胃的吸收，故药效增强。

炉　甘　石

【来源】本品为碳酸盐类矿石，主含碳酸锌（$ZnCO_3$）。

【炮制方法】

1. **炉甘石**　取原药材，除去杂质。

2. **煅炉甘石**　取净炉甘石，置耐火容器内，用武火加热，煅至红透后取出，立即投入水中浸淬，搅拌，倾取上层水中混悬液至烧杯或类似容器中，残渣继续煅淬3~4次，合并混悬液，静置数小时，待澄清后倾去上层清水，干燥。

3. **制炉甘石**　将药汁加入煅炉甘石细粉中拌匀，吸尽后干燥。药汁包括黄连汤，三黄汤（黄连、黄柏、黄芩）或五黄汤（黄连、黄柏、黄芩、栀子、大黄）。

每100kg煅炉甘石，均用各药12.5kg。

【炮制作用】

1. **炉甘石**　临床较少使用。

2. **煅炉甘石**　质地纯洁细腻，使用于外科及眼科外敷用。

3. **制炉甘石**　增强清热明目，敛疮收湿的作用。

第三节　闷煅法

1. 定义

药物在高温缺氧条件下煅烧成炭的方法。

2. 煅炭的目的

（1）产生或增强止血作用。如血余炭、棕榈炭。

（2）降低毒性。如干漆、蜂房。

3. 操作方法

将药物置于锅中，上盖一较小的锅，两锅结合处用砂或盐泥封严，扣锅上压一重物，用武火加热煅制成炭。

4. 注意事项

（1）煅炭防灰化。

（2）煅锅内药料放置适量，避免煅制不透。

（3）药物凉透后开锅。

5. 闷煅完成的检验方法

（1）滴水于盖锅底部即沸。

（2）扣锅底部贴张白纸，煅至纸呈深黄色即可。

（3）扣锅底部放几粒大米，煅至大米呈深黄色即可。

（4）两锅密封处裂隙冒出的烟雾由黑变白即可。

血　余　炭

【来源】本品是人头发制成的炭化物。

【炮制方法】

1. **头发**　取头发，除去杂质，用稀碱水洗净，清水漂净，晒干。

2. 血余炭　将洗净的头发装于大锅内，上扣一小锅，上压重物，两锅结合处用盐泥封固，武火煅制。

【炮制作用】

血余炭有止血作用。此药物作为止血丸在临床上用于各种出血症。

【炮制研究】

头发主含纤维蛋白，还含脂肪、铁、锌、铜、钙、镁等。煅炭后，其中的钙、铁元素的含量增高使得药物止血作用增强。药理实验结果也表明，血余炭有缩短凝血时间和收缩血管的作用。

棕　榈

【来源】本品为棕榈的干燥叶柄。

【炮制方法】

1. 棕榈　取原药材，除去杂质，切断。

2. 煅棕榈炭　将净棕榈装于大锅内，上扣一小锅，上压重物，两锅结合处用盐泥封固，武火煅制。

3. 炒炭　取净棕板，用武火炒至药材表面黑棕色，取出。

【炮制作用】

1. 棕榈　不生用。

2. 棕榈炭　具有止血作用。如治血崩不止的乌金散。

干　漆

【来源】本品来源于漆树树脂。

【炮制方法】

1. 煅干漆　将净干漆装于大锅内，上扣一小锅，上压重物，两锅结合处用盐泥封固，武火煅制。

2. 炒干漆　取净干漆，置锅中用武火炒至焦枯，烟尽。

【炮制作用】

1. 干漆　不生用。

2. 煅干漆　干漆煅后毒性与刺激性降低。具有破淤血、消积、杀虫的作用。如治恶血不行的干漆散。

【炮制研究】

干漆含漆酚可导致过敏性皮炎。经煅制后漆酚含量较低，刺激性作用下降，同时，干漆能缩短出血和凝血时间。

Chapter Eleven
Steaming, Boiling and Blanching

The method of steaming, boiling and blanching means preparing drugs with liquid and fire together. The "liquid" includes clean water, wine, vinegar or drugs' juice.

Section One   Steaming Method

1. Definition

It is a method that steams the drugs which are cut or purified with or without adjuvant materials (wine, vinegar or drugs juice) to some degree. The method of steaming in direct vapor is called 'Direct steam'. While steaming in a tightly closed container is called 'Indirect steam' or 'Stewing'.

2. Purposes

(1) Change drugs' nature and enlarge clinical usage. For example, the nature of the raw Radix Rehmanniae Recens (*Dihuang*) is cold. The effects are to remove heat and cool blood. After steaming, the nature changes from coldness to warmness, from bitterness to sweetness. The main effect changes from clearing to nourishing.

(2) Reduce side – effects. For example, after steaming, the cold and bitter nature of Radix et Rhizoma Rhei (*Dahuang*) could be moderated and the side effect of drastic purgation would be reduced.

(3) Remain efficacy and be good for storing. For example, after steaming, the eggs of Ootheca Mantidis (*Sangpiaoxiao*) would be killed so as to store.

(4) Facilitate softening of drugs. For example, Radix Scutellariae (*Huangqin*) should not be softened in cold water to avoid loss of effective components, it can be easily softened and cut after being steamed.

3. Operating Methods

The first method is to put drugs with or without adjuvant materials in steam container, steaming drugs to some degree.

The second method is to put drugs with liquid adjuvant materials, such as wine, in a closed container, steaming drugs to some degree.

4. Notice

1. The drugs steaming with liquid adjuvant materials should be steamed after the adjuvant materials being absorbed thoroughly.

2. The second method should be adopted when steaming drugs with liquid adjuvant materials.

3. The principle of steaming is 'strong fire first and then mild fire'.

4. In order to avoid drying out, drugs need to be steamed for a long time should keep adding hot water into the steam container.

5. Suitable Drugs

It is suitable for those drugs whose nature would be changed by steaming, especially the drugs that can nourish *yin* and tonify blood.

Radix Polygoni Multiflori (Heshouwu)

【Source】 Dry root.

【Processing Methods】

1. Raw Radix Polygoni Multiflori Remove impurities, clean, moisten drugs and cut them into thick pieces, then make them dry.

2. Steaming Radix Polygoni Multiflori Put drugs with soybean juice in a non – iron steam container, then steam until the decoction of black soybean is absorbed thoroughly by drugs and drugs show a brown color, take drugs out and dry. 10kg black soybean per 100kg drugs.

【Processing Functions】

1. Raw Radix Polygoni Multiflori It can remove toxicity for detumescence, and moisten dryness to relax bowels and check malaria. It is used for the dryness of the intestine and constipation, ulceration, swelling, itching and pain.

2. Steamed Radix Polygoni Multiflori After being steamed, it turns warm and sweet. It can tone up the liver and kidney, reinforce blood and essence, make beard and hair black and invigorate bones and muscles. For example, it can be used in Qibao Meiran Pills.

【Processing Research】

During steaming with soybean juice, the effect of diarrhea of Radix Polygoni Multiflori would be moderated because the component called anthraquinone could be transferred from combining type to liberation type with the extension of the steaming time. Meanwhile, the anti – aging effect of this drug would be enhanced because the contents of reducing sugar and lecithin increase after steaming. The study shows that the contents of reducing sugar in raw products and steaming products are 1.96% and 4.02% respectively, which means the decoction of black soybean has synergistic function.

Radix Scutellariae （Huangqin）

【Source】 Dry root.

【Processing Methods】

1. Raw Radix Scutellariae　Remove impurities, clean, steam drugs until the container full of vapour to make them soft and easy to be cut into small pieces.

2. Stir – frying Radix Scutellariae with Wine　Put drugs and wine together, mix them thoroughly. Add drugs into a preheated pot after the wine is absorbed thoroughly by drugs, then fry quickly with mild fire until drugs show a coke brown color and the natural flavor of adjuvant and drugs could be smelled, take drugs out and make them cool.

3. Charring Radix Scutellariae　Preheat the pot with high temperature, put drugs in and fry quickly until the drugs' outer color transforms to a coke brown color, and inner color turns yellow. Then take drugs out.

【Processing Functions】

1. Raw Radix Scutellariae　Make enzymes inactive and keep effective.

2. Radix Scutellariae stir – fried with Wine　It can conduct to upper energizer, clear away pathogenic fire, moderate the nature of bitterness and coldness, and avoid damaging splenic *yang*. For example, it can be used in Huangqin Xiefei Decoction which is suitable for conjunctival congestion.

3. Charred Radix Scutellariae　It can moderate the bitter and cold nature and strengthen the effect of hemostasis by clearing away heat. It is used for metrorrhagia, metrostaxis and vomit blood.

【Processing Research】

In order to be cut into small pieces, Radix Scutellariae Root should be softened by steaming rather than being soaked in cold water. Because the baicalin and wogonoside existing in raw products would be enzymolysised to baicalein and wogonin under suitable temperature and humidity, resulting the color of the drugs change from yellow to green when drugs are soaked in cold water.

After being stir – fried with wine, the bitter and cold nature of this drug would be moderated and the effect of clear heat could be conducted to upper energizer.

After being charred, the baicalin would be destroyed but the effect of hemostasis would show up because of the astringent nature of charred Radix Scutellariae.

Radix Rehmanniae Recens （Dihuang）

【Source】 Fresh or dried root tuber.

【Processing Methods】

1. Fresh Radix Rehmanniae Recens　Remove impurities of fresh drugs, cut them into thick pieces or wring juice.

2. Raw Radix Rehmanniae Recens　Remove impurities of the dried drugs. Soak drugs in the water until the outer color turns gray black and inner color turns yellowish brown. Cut drugs into thick pieces.

3. Prepared Radix Rehmanniae Recens（steaming with adjuvant materials）

Mix drugs with wine thoroughly and then put them in a closed container, steam above water until the wine is absorbed and the color turns black and drugs taste sweet, then cut drugs into thick pieces until the outer skin turns dry. 30 ~ 50kg wine per 100kg drugs.

4. Prepared Radix Rehmanniae Recens（steaming without adjuvant materials）

Put drugs in a closed container, steam drugs until they turn black, then make them eighty percent dry, and cut them into thick pieces.

5. Charring Radix Rehmanniae Recens
Preheat a pot with strong fire, put drugs in and fry quickly until the drugs' color shows burned black and start to swell, with bitter nature, take them out and make them cool.

6. Charring Prepared Radix Rehmanniae Recens
Preheat a pot with strong fire, put drugs in and fry quickly until the drugs' color turns burned black with sweet nature, take them out and make them cool.

【Processing Functions】

1. Fresh Radix Rehmanniae Recens
It can clear heat, promote fluid production, and cool blood to stop bleeding.

2. Raw Radix Rehmanniae Recens
It has bitter and cold nature. It can remove heat to cool blood, and nourish *yin* to promote the body fluid.

3. Prepared Radix Rehmanniae Recens
The nature changes from coldness to warmness, bitterness to sweetness, and the main effect transfers from clearing to nourishing. It has efficacy of nourishing *yin* and tonifying blood. For example, it can be used in Liuwei Dihuang Pills.

4. Charred Radix Rehmanniae Recens
Cool blood to stop bleeding.

5. Charred Prepared Radix Rehmanniae Recens
Nourish blood to stop bleeding.

【Processing Research】

The study shows that the contents of the extract of Radix Rehmanniae Recens are low but high in prepared Radix Rehmanniae Recens. The extract of ether shows the color of yellow in Radix Rehmanniae Recens and purple in prepared Radix Rehmanniae Recens. The contents of reducing sugar in prepared Radix Rehmanniae Recens are higher than those in Radix Rehmanniae Recens.

Section Two　Boiling Method

1. Definition

It means boiling drugs with or without adjuvant materials（solid adjuvant materials should be pounded or cut to pieces before boiling）in water to some degree.

2. Purposes

（1）Remove or decrease toxicity and side effects. For example, the toxicity of the raw Radix

Aconiti Preparata (*Chuanwu*) would be reduced after boiling. Boiling Sulfur (*Liuhuang*) with bean curd (200kg bean curd per 100kg sulfur) would reduce the toxicity and enhance the effect of warming kidney to invigorate *yang* and dejection.

(2) Change drugs' nature and strengthen effects. For example, after boiling with Radix Glycyrrhizae juice, the dryness of Radix Polygalae (*Yuanzhi*) would be moderated and the effect of calming the nerves and reinforcing intelligence would be strengthened.

(3) Clean drugs. For example, after boiling with bean curd, the grease of pearl would be removed and easy to use.

3. Operating Methods

Put drugs and clear water together, with or without adjuvant materials, heat drugs with strong fire at first and then keep boiling with mild fire to some degree.

The methods of boiling can be divided into three types, which include boiling without adjuvant materials, boiling with adjuvant materials (which can be divided into soaking in adjuvant materials first and then boiling, and decocting adjuvant materials first and then put drugs to boil together) , and boiling with bean curd.

4. Notice

(1) Remember to add suitable water when boiling.

(2) Keep boiling with mild fire.

(3) Before boiling, drugs should be separated by size to keep processing evenly and thoroughly.

(4) Dry timely after finishing boiling.

5. Suitable Drugs

It is suitable for toxic drugs or drugs which need to enhance effects, such as Radix Polygalae (*Yuanzhi*) , Margarita (*Zhenzhu*) .

6. Principle

Heat with strong fire at first and then keep boiling with mild fire.

Radix Aconiti Kusnezoffii (Caowu)

【Source】 Dry root tuber of Aconitum kusnezoffii Reichb.

【Processing Methods】

1. Raw Radix Aconiti Kusnezoffii　Take raw drugs, remove impurities.

2. Preparing Radix Aconiti Kusnezoffii　Soak drugs until no dryness inside, boil drugs in clear water until the inside of the drugs is not white in the big or solid ones and the drugs taste a little benumbed. Then cut drugs into thin pieces.

Before boiling, drugs should be separated by size. In order to inspect the soaking degree, the biggest one could be split to inspect the solid center. During processing, continuously add boiling water. Sometimes adjuvant materials also could be added to reduce the toxicity. The adjuvant materials include vinegar, licorice root, flos lonicerae and bean curd.

【Processing Functions】

1. Raw Radix Aconiti Kusnezoffii　It is toxic, external use only. It has the function of alleviating the swelling and stopping pain.

2. Prepared Radix Aconiti Kusnezoffii　After being processed, the toxicity reduced, and it can be used internally. For example, it can be used in Xiaohuoluo Pills which is suitable for cold – prevailing agonizing arthralgia.

【Processing Research】

After boiling, the drugs' toxicity could be reduced. The reason is that the toxic components are double ester aconitine. After being soaked in water, the part of such alkaloid would be decomposed. Meanwhile, heating would also make the double ester aconitine decompose into benzoyl aconitine whose toxicity is only $1/200 \sim 1/500$ of double ester aconitine, and then decompose into aconine whose toxicity is only $1/2000 \sim 1/4000$ of double ester aconitine.

The drugs should be soaked in water thoroughly after processing and then the water should be discarded.

Radix Polygalae （Yuanzhi）

【Source】 Dry root.

【Processing Methods】

1. Raw Radix Polygalae　Take raw drugs, remove impurities.

2. Stir – frying Radix Polygalae with Radix Glycyrrhizae (*Gancao*) juice　Mix drugs with licorice juice, heat with mild fire, and boil until the juice is absorbed by drugs thoroughly. 6kg licorice root per 100kg drugs.

Preparation of licorice juice　Boil Radix Glycyrrhizae two times. Condense the solution until the weight of juice is 10 times the weight of the original Radix Glycyrrhizae.

3. Stir – frying Radix Polygalae with honey　Put drugs and honey together with water diluting, mix them thoroughly. Put drugs into a preheated pot after honey is absorbed thoroughly by drugs, then fry quickly with mild fire till drugs become unstickly. 20kg honey per 100kg drugs.

【Processing Functions】

1. Raw Radix Polygalae　It is stimulating and for external use. Be used for superficial infection and swelling.

2. Stir – frying Radix Polygalae with licorice root juice　This method can moderate the dryness and remove numb nature of the drug. So it can calm the nerves and reinforce intelligence. For example, it can be used to treat forgetful insomnia in Yuanzhi Pills.

3. Stir – frying Radix Polygalae with honey　It can dissipate phlegm and stop cough. Especially used for the cough with excessive phlegm which is difficult to hawk.

【Processing Research】

According to the traditional processing method, the duramen of Radix Polygalae should be discarded while the root and the peel be chosen to make drugs. But the recent researches suggest that the drugs of peel and duramen have the same effects in toxicity, haemolyticus, calming mind and eliminating phlegm. So it is unnecessary to remove the duramen of the drug. Meanwhile, drugs prepared with licorice root juice could strengthen the effect of calming the nerves and reinforcing intelligence. Drugs prepared with honey could strengthen the effect of dissipating phlegm and stopping cough.

Section Three   Blanching Method

1. Definition

It means heating drugs in boiling water for a short time to separate seed coat and kernel.

2. Purposes

(1) Enhance effects. Take Semen Persicae (*Taoren*) for example.

(2) Separate different medicinal parts. Take Semen Lablab Album (*Baibiandou*) for example.

(3) Reduce toxicity. Take Semen Lablab Album for example.

3. Operating Methods

Boil plenty of clear water and put the drugs in. After several minutes, take them out immediately, and put into cold water as soon as possible, take them out, and knead to separate seed coat and kernel, screen out the coat.

4. Notice

(1) The amount of water should be more than ten times of the amount of drugs.

(2) Heat drugs till the outer part of the seed's coat changes from shrinking to expanding and easy to squeeze out the kernel.

(3) The time of blanching should be within short time, normally 5 to 10 minutes.

(4) During blanching, keep high temperature to prevent some effective components from being enzymolysised.

(5) Dry under the sun or use oven drying with low temperature.

Semen Armeniacae Amarum (Kuxingren)

【Source】 Dry and mature seed.

【Processing Methods】

1. Raw Semen Armeniacae Amarum Take raw drugs, remove impurities.

2. Blanching Semen Armeniacae Amarum Put drugs in boiled water for several minutes, take them out until the coat swell and put into cold water as soon as possible, and then knead to separate seed coat and kernel. The seed coat should be discarded and the kernel should be remained. Grind when used in clinical applications.

3. Stir – frying kernal of Semen Armeniacae Amarum Preheat with mild fire, and fry quickly until drugs' outer part shows yellowish with focal spots, take the drugs out and make them cool.

【Processing Functions】

1. Raw Semen Armeniacae Amarum It can direct *qi* downward to relieve cough and dyspnea and moisten dryness for relaxing bowels.

2. Stir – frying kernel of Semen Armeniacae Amarum The drugs' nature is warm after being stir – fried and will be good at warming lung for dispelling cold.

【Processing Research】

The purpose of blanching Semen Armeniacae Amarum is to make enzyme inactive to remain effective glycosides. The study shows that the content of hydrocyanic acid decreased after being processed, and thus the decrease of toxicity. Meanwhile, discarding no medicinal parts would help to prescribe in clinic. The study shows that the contents of effective components are 34.1% and 59.1% in apricot seed with coat and without coat respectively.

Semen Lablab Album （Baibiandou）

【Source】 Dry and mature seed.

【Processing Methods】

1. Raw Semen Lablab Album Take raw drugs, remove impurities.

2. Coat/kernel of Semen Lablab Album Put drugs into boiled water for several minutes, boiling until the coat become soften, then take drugs out of water and put in cold water, take them out, knead to separate seed coat and kernel. The bean coat and kernel both should be remained.

3. Stir – frying Semen Lablab Album Preheat a pot with mild fire, put drugs in and fry quickly until drugs' outer part shows yellowish with focal spots.

【Processing Functions】

1. Raw Semen Lablab Album It can invigorate stomach.

2. Coat of Semen Lablab Album It can dispel summer – heat and dissipate dampness.

3. Stir – frying Semen Lablab Album It has warm nature and can invigorate the spleen and stop diarrhea.

第十一章　蒸煮焯法

蒸、煮、焯法为"水火共制"法。这里的"水"可以是清水，也可以是酒、醋或药汁。

第一节　蒸　法

1. 定义

将净选或切制后的药物加辅料（酒、醋、药汁等）或不加辅料装入蒸制容器内隔水加热至一定程度的方法。直接利用流通蒸汽蒸者称为"直接蒸法"；药物在密闭条件下隔水蒸者称"间接蒸法"，又称"炖法"。

2. 蒸制的目的

（1）改变药性，扩大用药范围。如地黄生品性寒，清热凉血，蒸制后使药性转温，味道由苦转甜，功能由清变补。

（2）减少副作用。如大黄酒蒸后苦寒作用缓和，并能减轻腹痛等副作用。

（3）保存药效，利于储存。如桑螵蛸生品经蒸后杀死虫卵，便于储存。

（4）便于软化切片。如黄芩不能在冷水中软化，以免有效成分损失，蒸后便于软化切片。

3. 蒸制的操作方法

第一种方法是将药物加辅料或不加辅料放在蒸制容器内，用蒸汽加热蒸到一定程度的方法。

第二种方法是将药物加液体辅料，如酒，放置在密闭容器内用蒸汽加热到一定程度的方法。

4. 注意事项

（1）须用液体辅料拌蒸的药物应待辅料被吸尽后再蒸制。

（2）加液体辅料蒸制时必须采取第二种方法。

（3）蒸制时一般先用武火，再用文火。

（4）须长时间蒸制的药物宜不断添加开水，以免蒸汽中断。

5. 适用的药物

主要适用于通过蒸制可以改变性味的药物，特别是滋阴补血的药物。

何 首 乌

【来源】本品为何首乌的干燥根。

【炮制方法】

1. **何首乌**　取原药材，除去杂质，洗净，润透，切厚片，干燥。

2. **制何首乌**　取生首乌片，用黑豆汁拌匀，润湿，置非铁质容器内，密闭，蒸至药液吸尽，药物呈棕褐色时，取出，干燥。每100kg何首乌用黑豆10kg。

【炮制作用】

1. **何首乌**　具有解毒消肿、润肠通便、截疟的功能。用于肠道便秘，溃疡，肿胀，发痒和疼痛。

2. **制何首乌**　经蒸制后味转甘厚而性转温，增强了补肝肾、益精髓、乌须发、强筋骨的作用。如七宝美髯丸。

【炮制研究】

何首乌经黑豆汁蒸制过程中，结合蒽醌含量随蒸制时间的延长而减少，游离蒽醌的含量增加，使致泻作用减弱。同时，何首乌的抗衰老作用得到加强，因为还原糖和卵磷脂的含量蒸后增加。有研究表明，蒸制前和蒸制后何首乌还原糖的含量分别为1.96%和4.02%。说明黑豆汁有协调作用。

黄 芩

【来源】本品为黄芩的干燥根。

【炮制方法】

1. **黄芩**　取原药材，除去杂质，洗净。置蒸制容器内隔水加热，蒸至"圆汽"后，候软化后切薄片。

2. **酒黄芩**　取黄芩片，加黄酒拌匀，稍闷，待酒被吸尽后，用文火炒至表面微干，深黄色，嗅到辅料与药物的固有香气，取出，晾凉。

3. **黄芩炭**　取黄芩片，置热锅内用武火加热，炒至药物外面黑褐色，里面深黄色，取出。

【炮制作用】

1. **黄芩**　蒸后使酶灭活，保存药效。

2. **酒黄芩**　借黄酒升腾之力，清上焦肺热，同时，可缓和黄芩的苦寒之性，以免伤害脾阳。如治肺热咳嗽的黄芩泻肺汤。

3. **黄芩炭**　缓和了苦寒之性，以清热止血为主，用于崩漏下血，吐血衄血。

【炮制研究】

黄芩必须要蒸制软化，而不能用冷水处理，易变绿色。这是由于黄芩中的酶在一定温度和湿度下，可酶解黄芩中的黄芩苷和汉黄芩苷，产生黄芩素和汉黄芩素。

黄芩经酒制后，苦寒之性缓和，善清上焦热。

黄芩炒炭后，黄芩苷被破坏，且由于黄芩炭的吸附作用而产生了止血作用。

地 黄

【来源】 本品为地黄的新鲜或干燥根茎。

【炮制方法】

1. **鲜地黄** 取药材洗净，除去杂质，用时切厚片或绞汁。

2. **生地黄** 取干药材，除去杂质，用水闷润至外部灰黑色，内部黄褐色，切厚片。

3. **熟地黄（加辅料蒸制）** 取净生地，加黄酒拌匀，隔水蒸至酒吸尽，显乌黑色光泽，味转甜，取出，外皮稍干后切厚片。每100kg生地黄，用黄酒30~50kg。

4. **熟地黄（不加辅料蒸制）** 取净生地，蒸至黑润，取出，晒至八成干，切厚片。

5. **生地炭** 取生地片，武火炒至焦黑色，发泡鼓起，味苦时，取出放凉。

6. **熟地炭** 取熟地片，武火炒至外皮焦褐色，味甘，取出放凉。

【炮制作用】

1. **鲜地黄** 具有清热生津、凉血止血的功效。

2. **生地黄** 味甘，性寒。具有清热凉血、养阴生津的功效。

3. **熟地黄** 药性由寒转温，味由苦转甜，功能由清转补。具有滋阴补血、益精填髓的功能。如可用于六味地黄丸。

4. **生地炭** 凉血止血。

5. **熟地炭** 补血止血。

【炮制研究】

研究表明，熟地黄提取物含量高于生地黄。生地黄乙醚的提取物呈黄色，熟地黄呈紫色。熟地黄中还原糖的含量也高于生地黄。

第二节 煮 法

1. 定义

将净选过的药物加辅料或不加辅料放入锅内（固体辅料需先捣碎或切制），加适量清水同煮的方法。

2. 目的

（1）消除或降低药物的毒副作用。如川乌生品的毒性经煮制后明显降低。硫黄与豆腐同煮（每100kg净硫黄，用豆腐200kg）后，毒性降低，可增强助阳益火的作用。

（2）改变药性，增强药效。如远志用甘草水煮减其燥性，协同增强安神益智的功效。

（3）清洁药物。如珍珠经豆腐煮后可去其油腻，便于服用。

3. 操作方法

将药物加辅料或不加辅料放入锅内，加适量水，先用武火加热，煮沸后再用文火煮至一定程度。

煮法可分为3种，清水煮、加辅料煮（先加辅料闷润后煮和先加热辅料后投入药物共煮）、豆腐煮。

4. 注意事项

（1）煮制过程中及时补充水量。

（2）文火保持微沸。

（3）大小分档，分别炮制。

（4）煮好后出锅，及时烘干或晒干。

5. 适用的药物

适用于毒性药物或需增强药效的药物，如远志、珍珠。

6. 原则

武火煮至沸腾后，改用文火煎煮。

草　乌

【来源】本品为北乌头的干燥块根。

【炮制方法】

1. 生草乌　取原药材，除去杂质。

2. 制草乌　取净草乌，用水浸泡至内无干心，取出，加水煮沸至取大个及实心者切开内无白心，口尝微有麻舌感时，取出，切薄片。

煮制之前，药材必须大小个分开，以便观察浸泡的程度，大者浸泡至内无白心即可。煮制过程中需不断补充水量。也可加醋、甘草汁、金银花、豆腐等辅料降低其毒性。

【炮制作用】

1. 生草乌　有毒，仅做外用。具有消肿止痛的作用。

2. 制草乌　制后毒性降低，可供内服。如治寒湿痹痛的小活络丹。

【炮制研究】

草乌煮制之后，毒性降低。原因是其主要成分双酯型乌头碱在浸泡过程中被分解。同时，加热也使双酯型乌头碱水解为苯甲酰乌头胺，其毒性为双酯类乌头碱的 $1/200 \sim 1/500$。再进一步水解为乌头胺，其毒性为双酯类乌头碱的 $1/2000 \sim 1/4000$。

草乌须在水处理完全后，将处理的水弃去。

远　志

【来源】本品为远志的干燥根。

【炮制方法】

1. 远志　取原药材，除去杂质。

2. 甘草制远志　取甘草汁加入净远志，用文火煮至汤被吸尽，取出，干燥。每100kg 远志段，用甘草 6kg。

甘草汁制备： 取甘草，加适量水煎煮两次，合并煎液浓缩至甘草量的 10 倍。

3. **蜜炙远志** 取炼蜜，加适量开水稀释后，淋于远志段中，稍闷，用文火炒至蜜被吸尽，药色深黄，略带焦斑，疏散不黏手为度，取出，放凉。每 100kg 远志段，用炼蜜 20kg。

【炮制作用】

1. **远志** 有刺激性，多外用。用于表皮感染和消肿。

2. **甘草制远志** 缓和了燥性，消除了麻味，以安神益智作用为主。如治失眠健忘的远志丸。

3. **蜜炙远志** 增强化痰止咳的作用，多用于咳嗽，痰多，难咯出者。

【炮制研究】

远志传统加工方法要抽去木心，取根皮入药。现代研究表明，远志皮和远志木心在毒性、溶血、镇静和除痰作用上相近。所以，现认为远志没有去心的必要。同时，用甘草汁制可以增强益智安神的作用。蜜炙能增强化痰止咳的作用。

第三节 焯 法

1. **定义**

将药物置于沸水中浸煮短暂时间，取出，分离种皮的方法。

2. **目的**

（1）增强药效。如桃仁。

（2）分离不同的药用部位。如白扁豆。

（3）降低毒性。如白扁豆。

3. **操作方法**

先将多量清水加热至沸，再把药物投入沸水中，稍微翻烫数分钟，立即取出，浸漂于冷水中，捞起，搓开种皮、种仁，再筛去种皮。

4. **注意事项**

（1）水量一般为药量的 10 倍以上。

（2）药物要焯至种皮由皱缩到膨胀，易于挤脱时方可。

（3）焯制时间要短，一般为 5 ~ 10 分钟为宜。

（4）焯制过程中，温度要高，以防止药物有效成分被酶解。

（5）焯去皮后，宜晒干或低温烘干。

苦 杏 仁

【来源】本品为杏的干燥成熟种子。

【炮制方法】

1. **苦杏仁**　取原药材，除去杂质。

2. **燁杏仁**　取净杏仁置沸水中略煮，加热数分钟，至种皮膨胀捞起，用冷水浸泡，取出，搓开种皮与种仁，筛去种皮，用时捣碎。

3. **炒杏仁**　取燁杏仁，置锅内用文火炒至微黄色，略带焦斑，取出放凉。

【炮制作用】

1. **苦杏仁**　具有降气止咳平喘、润肠通便的功能。

2. **炒杏仁**　炒制后性温，长于温肺散寒。

【炮制研究】

燁苦杏仁的目的是杀酶保苷。研究表明，苦杏仁经加热炮制后，可以杀酶保苷，氢氰酸含量降低，故毒性降低。同时，除去了非药用部位，更利于临床调配处方。另有研究表明，苦杏仁去皮与不去皮药效成分所占的比例分别为 34.1% 和 59.1%。

白　扁　豆

【来源】本品为扁豆的干燥成熟种子。

【炮制方法】

1. **白扁豆**　取原药材，除去杂质。

2. **扁豆衣**　取净扁豆置沸水中，稍煮至皮软后，取出放凉水中稍泡，取出，搓开种皮与种仁，干燥，种皮和种仁均需保留。

3. **炒扁豆**　取净扁豆或仁，置热锅内，用文火炒至表面微黄，取出放凉。

【炮制作用】

1. **白扁豆**　具有健胃的作用。

2. **扁豆衣**　具有祛暑化湿的作用。

3. **炒扁豆**　炒后性温，偏于健脾止泻。

Chapter Twelve   Other Ways

Section One   Duplication Method

1. Definition

It refers to processing drugs repeatedly with several adjuvant materials.

2. Purposes

(1) Reduce or eliminate toxicity. For example, the ingredients of raw Rhizoma Pinelliae (*Banxia*) are toxic and irritant and can cause vomiting, so it is mostly used externally. After being processed by duplication methods, the toxicity and irritation could be moderated.

(2) Modify smell and taste. For example, the bad odor of Placenta Hominis (*Ziheche*) could be moderated by processing with wine and Pericarpium Zanthoxyli (*Huajiao*).

(3) Change the nature of drugs, improve drug efficacy or expand clinical application. For example, the nature of the products of raw Rhizoma Arisaematis (*Tiannanxing*) is pungent and warm, and its main function is removing cold phlegm. After being processed by bile, the warm nature becomes cold and the main function is to clear away heat phlegm.

3. Operating Method

Mix drugs with one or several adjuvant materials together, and process them by immersing in water or heating until the drugs get to the extent of regulation.

4. Feature

This method includes many procedures, so it often takes long time and asks for many adjuvant materials.

5. Suitable Drugs

Toxic drugs, such as Rhizoma Pinelliae (*Banxia*), Rhizoma Typhonii (*Baifuzi*), and Rhizoma Arisaematis (*Tiannanxing*).

Rhizoma Pinelliae (Banxia)

【Source】 Dry stem tuber.

【Processing Methods】

1. Raw Rhizoma Pinelliae Remove the impurities.

2. Preparing Rhizoma Pinelliae without adjuvant materials Add drugs with different sizes into alum solution separately, soak them and totally wet, and the cross sections show light grey with purple or white, and slight tongue numbing occurs. 20kg alum per 100kg drugs.

3. Preparing Rhizoma Pinelliae with ginger juice Soak drugs in water according to their sizes until the drugs are totally wet. Decoct fresh ginger to get the juice, then mix ginger juice, alum and drugs together. Boil them until they are thoroughly moistened, and the cross sections show yellowish white. 12.5kg alum and 25kg ginger per 100kg drugs.

4. Preparing Rhizoma Pinelliae with Radix Glycyrrhizae and lime water Soak drugs in water according to their sizes until totally wet. Decoct Radix Glycyrrhizae to get the juice, then mix the juice, lime water and drugs together. Soak drugs until the cross sections have a yellowish color and a kind of tongue numbing occurs. 15kg Radix Glycyrrhizae and 10kg calcined lime per 100kg drugs.

【Processing Functions】

1. Raw Rhizoma Pinelliae It is toxic and irritating, can cause vomiting, for external use.

2. Prepared Rhizoma Pinelliae without adjuvant materials It can moderate the nature of acridity and dryness and dry dampness to resolve phlegm. For example, it can be used in Erchen Decoction for cold phlegm cough.

3. Prepared Rhizoma Pinelliae with ginger juice It is warm and slightly dry, can warm the middle to eliminate phlegm and calm the adverse rise of *qi* to stop vomiting. For example, it can be used in phlematic vomiting – Xiaobanxia Decoction.

4. Prepared Rhizoma Pinelliae with Radix Glycyrrhizae and lime water It can eliminates cold phlegm, moderates the spleen and stomach. For example, it can be used in Xiangsha Yangwei Pills.

【Processing Research】

The researches show that after being processed, the toxicity of this drug would be reduced. The raw product has the highest content of toxicity, while the prepared Rhizoma Pinelliae without adjuvant materials and the prepared Rhizoma Pinelliae with ginger juice have lower content of such components. The studies also show that the effect of relieving vomiting and cough, and fighting tumors of Rhizoma Pinelliae prepared with Radix Glycyrrhizae and lime water is better than that of Rhizoma Pinelliae prepared without adjuvant materials.

Section Two Methods of Fermenting and Sprouting

1. Definition

It changes the nature of drugs, strengthens drug efficacy and produces new functions through fermenting and sprouting with catalysis and decomposition of enzyme.

2. Condition

(1) Fermenting condition: yeast, microbes, suitable temperature and dampness are needed.

(2) Sprouting condition: seed selection, suitable temperature, dampness and time are necessary. After fermenting or sprouting, most drugs need to be further processed.

Fermenting

1. Definition

It refers to the method that make drugs ferment or be purified with catalysis and decomposition of mold under suitable temperature and dampness.

2. Functions

(1) Produce new functions. For example, after being processed, the main effects of Massa Medicata Fermentata (*Liushenqu*) are invigorating spleens and improving appetite. The main effects of Medicinal Fermented Mass are promoting digestion, expelling wind – cold, invigorating spleens and regulating stomachs. The main effects of Semen Sojae Preparatum (*Dandouchi*) are relieving superficies and eliminating irritability.

(2) Change the nature of drugs and enhance drug efficacy. For example, after being processed, the main effects of Rhizoma Pinelliae fermented mass are invigorating spleens, warming stomachs, and drying dampness to resolve phlegm.

3. Special Condition

The suitable temperature and relative dampness for fermenting are 30℃ ~ 37℃ and 70% ~ 80% respectively. Other conditions include culture medium, pH 4 ~ 7.6, and enough oxygen or carbon dioxide.

4. Standard

The finished products should be yellowish white on their surfaces, spots inside, and fermented smell comes out. The black color and rancidity – odor should be avoided.

5. Notices

（1）Pre – process with anthelminthic and disinfection before fermenting is necessary.

（2）No interrupting during the process of fermentation.

（3）Pay attention to the temperature and humidity all the time during fermentation.

Massa Medicata Fermentata （Liushenqu）

【Source】 Fermented herbal mixture made of Semen Armeniacae Amarum （*Kuxingren*）, Semen Phaseoli （*Chixiaodou*）, fresh Herba Artemisiae Annuae （*Qinghao*）, fresh Fructus Xanthii （*Cangerzi*）, fresh Polygonum Hydropiper （*Laliao*） and flour.

【Processing Methods】

1. Massa Medicata Fermentata　Put all ingredients together and ferment them under suitable temperature and dampness. Take drugs out of the container and cut them into small pieces, then dry them and get the finished products. 4kg Semen Armeniacae Amarum and Semen Phasedi, 7kg fresh Herba Artemisiae Annuae, Polygonum Hydropiper and Fructus Xanthii per 100kg flour.

2. Stir – frying Massa Medicata Fermentata with bran　Heat the drugs with slow fire, stir – fry them quickly until the outer parts become yellowish or faint yellow. Preheating a pot with medium fire, put bran into the pot evenly. When smoke arises, add drugs in and stir – fry them quickly until drugs' outer parts show a claybank color. 10kg bran per 100kg drugs.

3. Parching Massa Medicata Fermentata　Preheat a pot with slow fire, then stir – fry the drugs quickly until the outer parts show a coke – brown color with coke aroma.

【Processing Functions】

1. Massa Medicata Fermentata　It can promote digestion and relieve superficies, used for food accumulation in stomach and intestine with fever caused by exogenous pathogens.

2. Stir – frying Massa Medicata Fermentata with bran　It is sweet and aroma, and the main effect are invigorate spleens, promote digestion and regulate the middle energizer.

3. Parched Massa Medicata Fermentata　It can promote digestion and resolve food stagnation, used for diarrhea caused by food stagnation.

Semen Sojae Preparatum （Dandouchi）

【Source】 Mature seed of black soybean.

【Processing Methods】

Decoct Folium Mori （*Sangye*） and Herba Artemisiae Annuae （*Qinghao*） together, soak soybeans in the decoction and boil them until the decoction is absorbed by soybeans thoroughly. Use the residue of decoction to cover the boiled soybean and ferment them for several days. Take fermented soybean out, clean and moist them for 15 ~ 20 days until fragrant aroma overflows. Dry them by steaming and the finished products can be obtained. 7 ~ 10kg Folium Mori and Herba Artemisiae Annuaeper 100kg drugs.

【Processing Functions】

Fermented Semen Sojae Preparatum are pungent, sweet and slightly bitter in flavor and cold in nature. It can relieve superficies and eliminate irritability, used for cold fever, dysphoria and sleep insufficiency.

【Processing Research】

There are still other adjuvant materials that can be used in soybean fermentation, including Folium Perillae (*Zisuye*) and Herba Ephedrae (*Mahuang*). The soybeans fermented with these two materials are pungent and warm in nature, while the soybeans fermented with Folium Mori (*Sangye*) and Herba Artemisiae Annuae (*Qinghao*) are pungent and cold in nature. Fermented soybeans processed with different materials have different clinical applications.

Sprouting

1. Definition

It refers to the method that make drugs sprout or be purified under suitable temperature and dampness.

2. Functions

After sprouting, starch in drugs can be decomposed into artificial gum, glucose and fructose; proteins can be decomposed into amino acids; fats can be decomposed to glycerin and fatty acids, meanwhile, digestive enzymes and vitamins will be produced. All these changes will make drugs produce new effects. For example, after sprouting, malt has the functions of promoting digestion, regulating stomach and delactation.

3. Special Condition

Before being chosen to sprout, the seeds should be given germination capacity tests. The germination capacity should be more than 85%. The standard of sprout length is 0.2cm. During sprouting, the suitable temperature is 18℃ ~ 25℃. Enough oxygen is necessary.

4. Processing Methods

Soak drugs in water under suitable temperature and dampness until they sprout, then dry them and get the finished products.

Fructus Hordei Germinatus (Maiya)

【Source】 Mature fruit of barley.

【Processing Methods】

1. Fructus Hordei Germinatus　Soak drugs whose germination capacity is more than 85% in water until they sprout. Take them out when the buds grow up to the length of 0.5 cm. Dry them and get the finished product.

2. Stir – frying Fructus Hordei Germinatus without adjuvant materials   Preheat a pot with slow fire, stir – fry the drugs quickly until the outer parts become deep yellow or claybank with nice smell.

3. Parching Fructus Hordei Germinatus   Preheat a pot with a medium fire, stir – fry the drugs quickly till they crack with both claybank or coke – brown colors on the outer parts and coke aroma.

【Processing Functions】

1. Fructus Hordei Germinatus   It is sweet in flavor and cool in nature. It can promote digestion, soothe liver stagnation and promoting flow of qi; used for dyspepsia, especially for rice, flour, and fruit stagnation; often used for heat produced by dyspepsia.

2. Stir – frying Fructus Hordei Germinatus without adjuvant materials   It is sweet in flavor and warm in nature. It can invigorate spleens to promote digestion.

3. Parched Fructus Hordei Germinatus   It is sweet and warm. It can promote digestion and food retention, especially for starch food retention, such as Sanxian Powder.

Section Three   Method of Making Frostlike Powder

1. Definition

It means making frostlike powder through degreasing, extracting, evaporating or decocting.

2. Suitable Drugs

Seeds, minerals and animal horns.

3. Notice

The method of heating and squeezing should be used for seeds' degreasing. Minerals should be processed in cool autumn days.

Making Frostlike Powder with Degreasing

1. Purpose

Reduce toxicity, moderate the nature of drugs and eliminate side effects. For example, the drastic purgation would be moderated after Fructus Crotonis (*Badou*) is defatted to powder.

2. Processing Method

Remove drugs' shell and get kernels, grind drugs to small pieces and wrap them with paper or cloth. After steaming, dry drugs in sunshine, squeeze and discard the paper or cloth, then repeat the procedure several times till get frostlike powder.

3. Notices

(1) After being processed, the paper or cloth should be discarded as soon as possible to avoid intoxication.

(2) During processing, heating is necessary.

(3) Content of grease should be 18% ~20% in defatted croton seed powder.

Fructus Crotonis (Badou)

【Source】 Dry and mature fruit of soybean.

【Processing Methods】

1. Raw Fructus Crotonis   Remove outer coats and get kernels.

2. Defatted Fructus Crotonis Seed Powder   Grind drugs to small pieces and wrap them with paper or cloth. After steaming, dry drugs in sunshine, squeeze and discard the paper cloth, then repeat the procedure several times until get frostlike powder.

【Processing Functions】

1. Raw Fructus Crotonis   It has strong toxicity, and used only externally. It can remove dyspeptic disease, fluid – purging and detumescent.

2. Defatted Fructus Crotonis Seed Powder   The toxicity is moderated, and it is used for ulcer, sore, swelling, and abdominal dropsy dilatation.

Making Frostlike Powder with Educing

1. Purpose

Make new drugs and improve drugs' efficacy.

Mirabilitum Praeparatum (Xiguashuang)

【Source】 Mature fruit of watermelon and Natrii Sulfas (*Mangxiao*).

【Processing Methods】

Cut fresh flesh of watermelons into small pieces, put one layer of fresh flesh with one layer of Natrii Sulfas on watermelon shells, and keep them until white crystals educe. 15kg Natrii Sulfas per 100kg watermelon.

【Processing Functions】

Ice watermelon has the effect of eliminating summer – heat, and Natrii Sulfas has the effect of clearing away heat and fire. The common action of the two drugs can make a new drug called Mirabilitum Praeparatum with the strong effect of purging away heat and fire.

Mirabilitum Praeparatum is always used in complex prescription, whose main effects are clearing away heat and relieving toxicity, eliminating inflammation to stop pain and bleeding. It is used for throat swelling and pain, and aphthae.

Making Frostlike Powder with Sublimating

1. Purpose

Purify drugs.

2. Processing Method

Put drugs in a big pot, and cover them with a small pot with heavy objects on. Seal the two pots with brine sludge or sand, calcined the drugs with high temperature, then collect the crystals that sublimate on the bottom of the small pot.

Arsenicum Sublimatum (Pishuang)

【Source】 Minerals containing arsenolite.

【Processing Methods】

1. Arsenicum Sublimatum　Discard impurities and grind drugs to fine powder.

2. White Arsenic　Put drugs in a big pot and cover them with a small pot with heavy objects on. Seal the two pots with brine sludge or sand, calcined with high temperature, then collect the crystals sublimating on the bottom of the small pot.

【Processing Functions】

1. Arsenicum Sublimatum　It can eliminate phlegm, stop coughing and expel parasites.

2. White Arsenic　It has more pure nature and stronger toxicity. For internal use, it can be used for eliminating phlegm, calming asthmas and checking malaria. For external use, it can be used for removing suppuration and anthelminthic.

Method of Making Frostlike Powder with Decocting

1. Purpose

Moderate the nature of drugs, expand clinical application and medicinal resource.

Cornu Cervi Degelatinatum (Lujiaoshuang)

【Source】 The lump or powder residue of the horn of Cervus nippon Temminck (*Meihualu*) or Cervus elaphus Linnaeas (*Malu*). After the glue is extracted, the residue is remained as Cornu Cervi Degelatinatum.

【Processing Methods】

Grind the lump or powder residues of the decocted horn of Cervus nippon Temminck or Cervus elaphus Linnaeas. The glue is extracted and the fine powder would be gotten.

【Processing Function】

It can warm kidney and tonify *yang*, and has the function hemostasis with astringent. For example, it can be used in Degelatined Deer – horn Pill and Degelatined Deer – horn Formula.

【Processing Research】

The hydrated calcium phosphate and calcium phosphate in this drug have the effect of astringent, thus strengthening the function of hemostasis.

Section Four   Methods of Roasting or Baking

1. Definition

It refers to the method that bakes purified or cut drugs with direct or indirect slow fire.

2. Purposes

(1) Make drugs easy to be stored and avoid mold.

(2) Make drugs easy to be crushed.

(3) Reduce toxicity of drugs.

3. Processing Method

Most drugs are roasted in baking oven or drying oven, while animal drugs are baked with direct fire. During processing, the heat level should be low and drugs need to be overturned continuously.

Tabanus （Mengchong）

【Source】 Dry feminal bodies of this insect.

【Processing Methods】

1. Raw Tabanus   Remove impurities, feet and wings.

2. Baking Tabanus   Bake drugs until drugs show yellowish brown or brownish black colors, and the texture becomes crisp.

3. Stir – frying Tabanus with rice   Preheat a pot with a medium fire, then put rice in evenly. Add drugs in when smoke occurs, and fry quickly until drugs' outer parts show a deep yellow color. 20kg rice per 100kg drugs.

【Processing Functions】

1. Raw Tabanus   It is slightly toxic, and has strong offensive smell of fish and drastic effect of activing blood.

2. Processed Tabanus   It has less toxicity and offensive smell of fish, and is easier to be crushed, which makes it less stimulating to stomach. It can be used for blood stasis and injury from fall.

Scolopendra （Wugong）

【Source】 Dry whole bodies of this insect.

【Processing Methods】

1. Raw Scolopendra　Remove impurities, feet and wings.

2. Baking Scolopendra　Bake drugs with low heat until they become dark brown and the texture becomes crisp.

【Processing Functions】

1. Raw Scolopendra　It has pungent and warm nature with toxicity. It can relieve spasms and extinguish wind, used for infantile convulsions and tetanus.

2. Baked Scolopendra　The toxicity of the drug could be reduced after being baked. It has moderated smell and taste and is easier to be crushed. Same functions as the raw drugs.

Section Five　Method of Roast in Fresh Cinders

1. Definition

It refers to the method that wraps drugs with wet paper or flour, and puts them in heated clam powders or bran to remove some grease.

2. Purposes

Reduce the side – effects of drugs, moderate their medical nature and enhance their efficacy.

3. Classification

Roasting methods include roasting with bran, flour, talcum powder, paper or wet paper.

4. Notices

During roasting, we should pay attention to the differences between roasting and stir – frying with adjuvant materials. Take roasting with bran and stir – frying with bran for examples, for the dosage of adjuvant materials, the former ratio is 100 : 40, and the latter is 100 : 10 ~ 100 : 15. For the fire power and time, the former should be processed with a low fire and last for relatively long time, and the latter should be processed with medium fire for less time. The operation procedure: the former asks for putting drugs and bran in a container together at the same time, and the latter asks for heating bran first and then adding drugs in a container.

Semen Myristicae (Roudoukou)

【Source】Dry seeds.

【Processing Methods】

1. Roasting Semen Myristicae with Bran　Heat drugs and bran together with slow fire, stir them constantly until drugs become deep brown and bran becomes light yellow. 40kg bran per 100kg drugs.

2. Roasting Semen Myristicae with Talcum Powder   Preheat talcum powder until it flows freely, then add drugs in with constant stirring until drugs become deep brown with strong aroma, 50kg talcum powder per 100kg drugs.

3. Roasting Semen Myristicae with Flour Wrap   Wrap nutmeg with flour, preheat talcum powder until it flows freely, add drugs in and stir them constantly until the flour becomes yellow. 50kg flour is used for every 100kg drugs.

【Processing Functions】

1. Semen Myristicae   It contains oil. It can irritate intestine, and has the effect of warming stomach to remove food stagnation, descending *qi* to stop vomiting.

2. Roasted Semen Myristicae with Bran/Talc powder/Flour   The side effects of diarrhea is moderated and the function of antidiarrhea with astringent is strengthened.

Section Six   Method of Defecating

1. Definition

It means purifying some minerals, especially soluble inorganic salt minerals through the procedure of dissolving, filtering and recrystallization.

2. Purposes

(1) Purify drugs and enhance efficacy.

(2) Alter the nature of drugs.

(3) Reduce the toxicity of drugs.

3. Processing Methods

(1) Lower the temperature for crystallizing (cold crystallizing). Boil drugs and adjuvant materials together, then filter them. Put the filtrate in a shady and cool place to make them become cool, collect the crystals.

(2) Evaporate for crystallizing (hot crystallizing). Heat drugs and water together until drugs dissolve, filter and collect the filtrate, mix vinegar with the filtrate until the water evaperated. Then the crystals are educed on the surface of the filtrate, collect the crystals.

Natrii Sulfas (Mangxiao)

【Source】   Crystals containing Natrii Sulfas with water of hydration.

【Processing Methods】   Boil drugs and turnips together, then filter them and collect the filtrate. Put the filtrate in a shady and cool place to make them cool and collect the crystals. Every 20kg turnip needs 100kg drugs. The suitable temperature of processing is $2℃ \sim 4℃$.

【Processing Functions】

1. Mirabilite It can expel pathogenic heat to loosen bowels, moisten dryness and soften hardness.

2. Natrii Sulfas It can moderate the cold and salty properties, strengthen the effect of removing stagnation and lowering adverse – rising energy.

Sal Ammoniac (Naosha)

【Source】 Crystals containing sodium chloride.

【Processing Methods】

Heat drugs and water together until drugs dissolve, filter the mixture and collect the filtrate. Mix vinegar with the filtrate, evaporate water and the crystals will be formed on the surface of the filtrate, then collect the crystals. 50kg vinegar per 100kg drugs. The suitable temperature of processing is 80℃.

【Processing Functions】

1. Raw Sal Ammoniac It can remove stagnation and soften hardness, causticity and external use only.

2. Sal Ammoniac processed with Vinegar It is pure with less toxicity. It has the effect of removing stagnation and softening hardness.

Section Seven Grinding Drugs in Water

1. Definition

It refers to preparing fine powder of drugs which are insoluble in water through grinding drugs in water repeatedly according to different floating property of coarse and fine powder.

2. Purposes

(1) Remove impurities and clean drugs.

(2) Make drugs exquisite.

(3) Avoid dust flying up during grinding.

(4) Reduce toxicity.

3. Processing Method

Grinding drugs with water for several minutes, add more water in and get the suspension, and pour out the suspension into another container. The remainder will be processed in the same way for several times. Suspension is collected and kept still for some time. Then the precipitate is collected and the supernatant is discarded.

4. Notices

(1) Less water during grinding.

(2) More water during stirring to get the suspension.

(3) Open – air drying and avoid heating.

(4) Avoid iron when grinding cinnabar and realgar.

5. Suitable Drugs

It is suitable for drugs being insoluble in water, such as realgar, cinnabar and pearl.

Cinnabaris (Zhusha)

【Source】Minerals containing mercuric sulfide.

【Processing Methods】

Grinding drugs with water for several minutes, add more water in and get the suspension, and pour the suspension in another container. The remainder will be processed in the same way for several times. Collect the suspension, keep it still for some time, collect the precipitate and discard the supernatant.

【Processing Functions】

Cinnabar has the effect of inducing sedation, tranquilization and detoxifying. After being processed, the drugs are easy to be used in preparation.

Section Eight   Method of Dry Distillation

1. Definition

It refers to baking or burning drugs in a container to produce pyrolysate.

2. Purposes

Produce new pyrolysate that is different from original drugs for clinical use.

3. Processing Methods

(1) Collect from the upper part, that is to collect condensate. For example, Pityrolum (*Heidouliuyou*) would be collected by this method.

(2) Collect from the lower part, that is to collect liquid from drugs directly. For example, juice of bamboo. Succus Bambusae would be collected by this method.

(3) Collect by stir – frying, that is to collect the oily materials. For example, egg oil would be collected by this method.

Phyllostachyl nigra（Lodd. ex Lindl.）
Munro var. henonis（Mitf.）Stapf et Rendle（Zhuli）

【Source】 Pyrolysate of henon bamboo.

【Processing Methods】

Collect the liquid from the lower part from drugs directly. The processing temperature is 350℃ ~400℃.

【Processing Functions】

It has the functions of clearing away heat and phlegm, relieving convulsions and promoting defecation.

Yolk Oil（Danhuangyou）

【Source】 Oil of eggs.

【Processing Methods】

Collect oily materials by stir – frying egg yolk, evaporate water as far as possible with slow fire and then decoct the grease with high heat（280℃）.

【Processing Functions】

It has the functions of antimycotic and ananaphylaxis.

Black Soyabean Tar（Heidouliuyou）

【Source】 Oil of black soybean.

【Processing Methods】

Collect the condensate from the upper part. The processing temperature is 400℃ ~450℃.

【Processing Functions】

It has the functions of clearing away heat, eliminating dampness and diminishing inflammation.

第十二章　其他方法

第一节　复　制　法

1. 定义

用数种辅料反复炮制药物的方法。

2. 目的

（1）减少或除去毒性成分。例如，生半夏所含成分是有毒的并具有刺激性，会至呕吐，所以常常外用。使用复制法炮制后，其毒性和刺激性有所减轻。

（2）矫臭矫味。例如，紫河车用酒和花椒炮制后，除去了腥臭味。

（3）改变药物性质，增强药物疗效或者扩大临床应用。例如，生天南星所含成分的性质是辛温的，主要功效是消除寒痰。用胆汁炮制后，性由温转寒，主要功效是清除热痰。

3. 操作方法

将药物放入一种或数种辅料中，通过水浸或加热处理，直到药物达到规定的程度。

4. 特点

此方法包含许多过程，因此花费时间较长，用到辅料较多。

5. 适宜的药物

有毒药物，如半夏 、白附子、天南星。

半　　夏

【来源】本品为半夏的干燥块茎。

【炮制方法】

1. **半夏**　除去杂质。

2. **清半夏**　将大小分档的药物加到白矾溶液中，浸泡至内无干心，横切面呈浅灰而带紫红色或者白色，微有麻舌感。每100kg半夏，用白矾20kg。

3. **姜半夏**　取净半夏，大小分档，用水浸泡至内无干心，取新鲜生姜煎汁，将姜汁、明矾、药物一起煎煮至透心，断面呈黄白色。100kg 半夏，用明矾 12.5kg 和生姜 25kg。

4. **法半夏** 取净半夏，大小分档，用水浸泡至内无干心，取甘草煎汁，将甘草汁、石灰水和药物一起浸泡至断面呈黄色，微有麻舌感时取出。100kg 半夏，用甘草 15kg、生石灰 10kg。

【炮制作用】

1. **半夏** 有毒，并具有刺激性，致呕，常外用。

2. **清半夏** 缓和了辛燥之性，具有燥湿化痰之效，如治疗寒痰咳嗽的二陈汤煎剂。

3. **姜半夏** 性温微燥，具有温中祛痰、降逆止呕之效，如治疗痰饮呕吐的小半夏汤。

4. **法半夏** 祛寒痰，调和脾胃，如香砂养胃丸。

【炮制研究】

研究表明，炮制后，半夏毒性降低。生半夏所含毒性成分最高，清半夏和姜半夏所含毒性成分最低。研究还表明，法半夏的镇咳镇呕和抗肿瘤效果比清半夏要好。

第二节　发酵、发芽法

1. 定义

借助酶的分解和催化作用，使药物发芽和发酵，从而达到改变药物性质，增强和产生新的功效。

2. 条件

（1）发酵条件：酵母，微生物，适宜的温度和湿度。

（2）发芽条件：选种，适宜的温度、湿度和时间，发芽或发酵后，大部分药物需要进一步炮制处理。

一、发酵

1. 定义

在适宜的温度和湿度下，利用霉菌催化分解，使药物发泡或纯化的方法。

2. 作用

（1）产生新的疗效。例如，六神曲经炮制后，具有健脾和促进食欲的作用。建神曲的主要功效是促进消化，祛除风寒，健脾和胃。淡豆豉的主要功效是解表除烦。

（2）改变药物性质，增强药物疗效。例如，炮制后，半夏曲的主要功效为健脾暖胃，燥湿化痰。

3. 专属条件

发酵的适宜温度是 30℃ ~ 37℃，相对湿度是 70% ~ 80%，其他条件还包括培养基，

pH 值 4 ~ 7.6，足够的氧气或者二氧化碳。

4. 标准

成品表面黄白色，内部有斑点，同时带有酵香气味。不应出现黑色及酸败味。

5. 注意事项

（1）药物在发酵前要先进行杀虫、杀菌处理。
（2）发酵过程不能中断。
（3）发酵过程要时刻注意温度和湿度。

六　神　曲

【来源】为苦杏仁、赤小豆、鲜青蒿、鲜苍耳、鲜辣蓼和面粉发酵成的曲剂。

【炮制方法】

1. 六神曲　把所有成分放在一块，在适宜的温度和湿度下进行发酵，取出药物，切成小块，干燥，即得最后的炮制品。每100kg 面粉，用苦杏仁、赤小豆各4kg，鲜青蒿、鲜辣蓼、鲜苍耳各7kg。

2. 炒/麸炒六神曲　文火加热，快速翻炒，至药物表面呈黄色或淡黄色；或用中火加热锅，将麦麸倒进锅里，当有烟产生时，加入药物快速翻炒，直到药物表面呈棕黄色。每100kg 药物，用10kg 麦麸。

3. 焦六神曲　用文火预热锅，快速翻炒直到药物表面呈焦褐色。

【炮制作用】

1. 六神曲　具有消食解表的作用，用于治疗食积不化兼外感发热。

2. 麸炒六神曲　具有甘香气，以健脾、消食和中为主。

3. 焦六神曲　消食化积力强，治食积泄泻为主。

淡　豆　豉

【来源】黑豆的成熟种子。

【炮制方法】

将桑叶和青蒿一起煎煮，将大豆放到煎液中，煮沸直到汤液被大豆吸尽，用煮过的桑叶和青蒿覆盖煮过的大豆，发酵几天。取出淡豆豉，去除杂质，闷15 ~ 20 天直到有香气逸出，蒸干，即得淡豆豉。每100kg 黑大豆，用桑叶、青蒿各7 ~ 10kg。

【炮制作用】

淡豆豉，味辛、甘、微苦，性寒。能解表除烦，用于寒冷发热、烦躁不安和睡眠不足。

【炮制研究】

另有一些其他的辅料，可以用在大豆发酵中，包括紫苏叶和麻黄。例如，由这两种材料制成的大豆黄卷，其性质辛温，而由桑叶和青蒿草发酵而成的淡豆豉，其性质是辛寒，因此，这两个发酵大豆因加工材料不同，而有不同的临床应用。

二、发芽

1. 定义

在适宜温度和湿度条件下，使药物提纯或发芽的方法。

2. 作用

经过萌芽，药物中淀粉可以被分解为糊精、葡萄糖及果糖；蛋白质可以被分解为氨基酸；脂肪可以被分解为甘油和脂肪酸，同时，会产生消化酶和维生素。所有这些变化将使药物产生新的效果。例如，经过发芽，麦芽具有促进消化、调和胃和回奶的作用。

3. 专属条件

在发芽前应通过发芽能力测试，要求发芽率在85%以上。芽的长度为0.2cm的标准。发芽的适宜温度为18℃~25℃。足够的氧气是必要的。

4. 炮制方法

在合适的温度和湿度下，将药物浸在水中直到发芽，干燥，得到成品。

麦　芽

【来源】大麦的成熟果实。

【炮制方法】

1. **麦芽**　选取发芽力超过85%的麦子浸泡在水中，直到发芽，待芽的长度长到0.5cm取出，干燥，得到成品。

2. **炒麦芽**　用文火将锅预热，迅速翻炒，直到药物的表面呈深黄色或棕黄色，有香气。

3. **焦麦芽**　先用中火预热锅，快速翻炒至爆裂，药物的表面呈棕黄色或焦黑色，且具焦香味。

【炮制作用】

1. **麦芽**　味甜，性凉，有促进消化、疏肝解郁和行气的作用。用于消化不良，尤其是大米、面粉、水果引起的停滞。常用于食积化热。

2. **炒麦芽**　味甘性温，健脾消食。

3. **焦麦芽**　味甜，性温，促进食物消化，尤其是淀粉引起的食积。例如，三仙散。

第三节　制　霜　法

1. 定义

透过除油、提取、蒸发或煎煮法制得松散粉末的方法。

2. 适合的药材

种子、矿物质、动物的角。

3. 注意事项

种子应该用加热和挤压方法进行去油。矿物质制霜最好在秋天进行。

一、去油制霜法

1. 目的

降低毒性，缓和药性，降低副作用。例如，巴豆经去油制霜后，其峻猛的泻下作用得到缓和。

2. 炮制方法

除药物的外壳，取得的内核，将药物研细，用纸或布包裹。蒸后，将药物放在阳光下晒干，榨去油并弃去纸或包布，如此重复数次，直到药物松散成粉。

3. 注意事项

（1）药物经过处理后，所用的纸或布应该尽快丢弃，以避免中毒。
（2）在处理过程中，必须进行加热。
（3）巴豆霜的油脂含量应为 18% ~ 20% 。

巴　　豆

【来源】本品为大豆的干燥成熟种子。
【炮制方法】
1. 巴豆　除去外衣，得到种核。
2. 巴豆霜　将药物研细，用纸或布包裹。蒸后，将药物放在阳光下晒干，榨去油，如此重复数次，直到药物松散成粉。
【炮制作用】
1. 巴豆　毒性强，仅外部使用。促进消化，逐水消肿。
2. 巴豆霜　毒性降低，用于溃疡，疮痈肿胀，腹水膨胀。

二、渗析制霜法

1. 目的
制造新药，增加药物疗效。

西　瓜　霜

【来源】西瓜的成熟果实和芒硝。

【炮制方法】

将新鲜的西瓜肉切成小块，在空西瓜壳里填上芒硝，用新鲜西瓜肉和芒硝覆盖，直到有白色结晶产生。每100kg 西瓜，用15kg 芒硝。

【炮制作用】

冰西瓜具有除暑热作用，芒硝具有清热降火作用。这两种药物共制产生一种新药西瓜霜，具有很强的清热泻火作用。

西瓜霜常用在复方中，主要作用是清热解毒，消炎止痛，止血。用于咽喉肿痛、口舌生疮等。

三、升华制霜法

1. 目的

纯净药物。

2. 炮制方法

将药物放在一大锅中，上面扣一小锅，小锅上加重物，结合处用盐泥或砂土封固，高温煅烧，收集盖锅上的升华结晶。

砒　　霜

【来源】含有砒石的矿物质。

【炮制方法】

1. **信石**　去除杂质，研细。

2. **砒霜**　将药物放在一大锅中，上面扣一小锅，小锅上加重物，结合处用盐泥或砂土封固，高温煅烧，收集盖锅上的升华结晶。

【炮制作用】

1. **信石**　祛痰、止咳和驱虫。

2. **砒霜**　药性更纯，毒性更强。内服可以祛痰平喘、截疟；外用具有祛腐、杀虫的功效。

四、煎煮制霜法

1. 目的

缓和药性，扩大临床应用，扩大药源。

鹿　角　霜

【来源】由梅花鹿或马鹿的角煎煮成的角块或粉渣，胶状物需要被提纯，取其残留物。

【炮制方法】

将梅花鹿或马鹿的角煎煮成的角块或粉渣研细，将胶状物提纯，得细粉。

【炮制作用】

温肾补阳，收敛止血。例如，鹿角霜丸和鹿角霜方。

【炮制研究】

鹿角霜中所含的含水磷酸钙和磷酸钙具有收敛止血作用，这就增强了其止血功能。

第四节　烘 焙 法

1. 定义

将净选或切制后的药物用文火直接或间接烘干的方法。

2. 目的

（1）使药物便于贮存，避免发霉。
（2）使药物易于粉碎。
（3）降低药物毒性。

3. 炮制方法

一般的药物用烘箱或者干燥箱进行烘焙，动物类药物要用直火进行烘焙，在炮制过程中用文火，并要不断的翻动药物。

虻 虫

【来源】雌性的干燥全体。

【炮制方法】

1. **虻虫**　除去杂质和足翅。

2. **烘虻虫**　用火焙药，直到药物表面呈棕黑色或黄褐色，质地酥脆时为止。

3. **米炒虻虫**　用中火预热锅，加入米，炒到冒烟时投入药物，不断翻炒直到药物表面呈深黄色。每100kg虻虫用米20kg。

【炮制作用】

1. **虻虫**　有小毒，有腥臭味，具有很强的活血作用。

2. **制虻虫**　降低毒性和腥臭味，降低对胃的刺激作用，便于粉碎，用于血瘀经滞，跌打损伤。

蜈 蚣

【来源】干燥全体。

【炮制方法】

1. **蜈蚣**　除去杂质和足翅。

2. **焙蜈蚣**　用文火烘焙直到药物呈黑褐色，质地变脆为止。

【炮制作用】

1. **蜈蚣**　辛温，有毒，具有息风平痉的作用，用于小儿惊风和破伤风。

2. **焙蜈蚣**　降低毒性，矫臭矫味，易于粉碎，与原药材有相同的功效。

第五节 煨 法

1. 定义

将药物用湿纸或湿面粉包裹，放到加热的蛤粉或麦麸中，除去部分油脂的方法。

2. 目的

减少副作用，缓和药性，增强疗效。

3. 分类

煨法可以分为麦麸煨，面粉煨，滑石粉煨，纸或湿纸煨。

4. 注意事项

在煨法中，要注意辅料煨和辅料炒之间的不同。例如，麦麸煨和麦麸炒，需辅料量，在麦麸煨中，每100kg药材，用麦麸40kg，而在麦麸炒中，每100kg药材，用麦麸10～15kg；所用的火候，麦麸煨法中要用文火，炮制时间相对较长，麦麸炒法中用中火，炮制时间短；操作步骤，麦麸煨法，药物和麦麸同时放到锅里，麦麸炒，先加热麦麸，再投入药物。

肉 豆 蔻

【来源】干燥种子。

【炮制方法】

1. 麦麸煨 将药物和麦麸一起用文火加热，不断翻动，直到药物表面呈深棕色，麦麸呈浅黄色。每100kg药物，用麦麸40kg。

2. 滑石粉煨 将滑石粉反复预热，直到呈灵活状态，投入药物，不断翻动，直到药物呈深棕色，有浓香。每100kg药物，用滑石粉50kg。

3. 面粉煨 用面粉将药物包裹，将滑石粉置锅内炒至灵活状态，投入药物，不断翻动，直到面粉呈黄色。每100kg药物，用面粉50kg。

【炮制作用】

1. 肉豆蔻 含有油脂，刺激肠道，具有暖胃消食、下气止呕的作用。

2. 煨肉豆蔻 降低滑肠副作用，增强了固肠止泻的功能。

第六节 提 净 法

1. 定义

通过溶解、过滤、重结晶的方法提纯一些矿物质类药物，特别是含有不溶的无机盐的矿物质类药物。

2. 目的

（1）纯化药物，增加疗效。
（2）改变药物性质。
（3）减低毒性。

3. 炮制方法

（1）降温结晶（冷结晶）。将药物与辅料共煮后，过滤，将滤液置阴凉处，使之冷却，收集结晶。
（2）蒸发结晶（热结晶）。将药物与水共热直到药物溶解，过滤，收集滤液，在滤液中加醋混合，把水分蒸干，在滤液表面有结晶生成，收集结晶。

芒　硝

【来源】含水芒硝的结晶。
【炮制方法】
将药物与萝卜共煮，滤过，收集滤液，放置阴凉处，待冷却后收集结晶，每100kg药物，用萝卜20kg。炮制的适宜温度是2℃～4℃。
【炮制作用】
1. **朴硝**　泻热通便，润燥软坚。
2. **芒硝**　缓和寒咸之性，增强了消导降气之功。

硇　砂

【来源】氯化钠结晶。
【炮制方法】
将药物与水共热直到药物溶解，过滤，收集滤液，在滤液中加醋混合，把水分蒸干，在滤液表面有结晶生成，收集结晶。每100kg药物，用醋50kg。炮制的适宜温度是80℃。
【炮制作用】
1. **硇砂**　消滞，软坚，具有腐蚀性，仅外用。
2. **醋制硇砂**　纯化药物，降低毒性，增强消滞软坚的作用。

第七节　水　飞　法

1. 定义

利用粗细粉末在水中悬浮度不同，将不溶于水的药物与水反复研磨，分离得到细粉的方法。

2. 目的

（1）除去杂质，洁净药物。
（2）使药物质地细腻。
（3）在研磨过程中防止粉尘飞扬。
（4）降低毒性。

3. 炮制方法

将药物与水研磨数分钟，再加水，使悬浮，倒出悬浮液，剩余部分再进行研磨，如此反复操作，使收集悬浮液静置，去掉上面的水，收集沉淀。

4. 注意事项

（1）在研磨时，水量应少。
（2）搅拌时水量宜大。
（3）晾干，不宜加热。
（4）研磨朱砂和雄黄时要忌铁器。

5. 适宜的药物

不溶于水的药物，如雄黄、朱砂、珍珠。

朱　　砂

【来源】含硫化汞的矿物质。
【炮制方法】
将药物与水研磨数分钟，再加水，使悬浮，倒出悬浮液，剩余部分再进行研磨，如此反复操作，使收集悬浮液静置，去掉上面的水，收集沉淀。
【炮制作用】
朱砂具有镇静安神、解毒的作用。经炮制后，易于制剂。

第八节　干馏法

1. 定义

将药物置于容器中焙烤使其产生干馏物的方法。

2. 目的

制备有别于原药材的干馏物，以适合临床需要。

3. 炮制方法

（1）上部收集。收集冷凝液，例如，黑豆馏油。

（2）下部收集。收集液体，例如，竹沥油。

（3）炒制收集。收集油类物质，例如，蛋黄油。

竹　沥

【来源】淡竹的干馏物。

【炮制方法】

收集下部液体，炮制温度为350℃~400℃。

【炮制作用】

清热痰，抗惊厥，促进排便。

蛋　黄　油

【来源】蛋黄的油。

【炮制方法】

通过炒制，收集油类物质。用文火使水分尽量蒸发，然后用武火煎出油（280℃）。

【炮制作用】

抗过敏和抗真菌。

黑豆馏油

【来源】黑豆的油。

【炮制方法】

收集上部冷凝液，炮制温度为400℃~450℃。

【炮制作用】

清热，利湿，消炎。